ESSENTIAL OILS
A Concise Guide

J. A. von Fraunhofer
MSc, PhD, FASM, FADM, FRSC
Professor Emeritus
Health Sciences Center
University of Maryland

ISBN-13: 978-1975845735
ISBN-10: 1975845730

DEDICATION

This book is dedicated to my wife, Susan, without whom none of
this would be worth it.

CONTENTS

PREFACE

As someone who likes to cook and a lover of good food, I am familiar with flavors and flavoring and that good cooks rely on the cooking process to extract essential oils from spices.[a] However, probably like most people, fragrances and perfumes are very much a "black art" to me. It came as a major surprise, for example, when I recently learned that the distinctive smell and flavor of liquorice (a smell and taste that some people love and others loathe) have been identified as due to the presence of 39 aroma compounds.[b] The scientific finding that numerous aroma-active compounds contribute to the smell and taste of liquorice undoubtedly is also the case for virtually every other plant or vegetable that possesses a distinctive odor or taste. Obviously, aroma is a far more complex and intriguing scientific subject than I had ever suspected.

That the wavelengths of light and the frequency of sound waves determine the colors recognized by the eye and the pitches perceived by the ear are the sounds we hear are well understood, but little is known about the sense of smell. Science refers to the sense of smell as the olfactory system and virtually every human, animal and a good many avian species possess a sense of smell, but there is a wide divergence in the olfactory capabilities of living creatures. The main function of the olfactory system is to detect, perceive and

---

[a] J. A. von Fraunhofer. Vitamins, Minerals and Spices. Kindle/CreateSpace, Seattle, WA (2013).
[b] Secret of liquorice smell unraveled; Chemistry World (2017) 14 (1): 50; J. Wagner, M. Granvogl and P. Schieberle; J. Agric. Food Chem. (2016).

identify the chemicals that are floating in the air. Apparently when we sniff something, the mucus membranes in the nose dissolve the chemicals from the air and these molecules are then carried to the olfactory receptors in the brain. That is what we "smell".

Whereas skilled testers often can distinguish between near-identical smells, there is no reliable or accurate method of predicting how humans will characterize the smell or aroma of a particular molecule. What complicates the issue is that molecules with completely different structures and compositions can have near identical aromas. Clearly the aroma or smell of essential oils is a large and very complex subject and may be highly individualized regarding what people like or dislike, a phenomenon recognized by perfume manufacturers when they produce their cosmetics.

Given the evocative effects of liberated essential oils from plants, it is unsurprising that there is a major, and growing, interest in the mental and physical health benefits of experiencing pleasing and satisfying scents – what is known as aromatherapy. In addition to aromatherapy, there are growing numbers of products based on essential oils that provide numerous overall mental and physical health benefits for their users. The objective of this book is to provide the reader with a concise, understandable and readable guide to essential oils. It discusses what they are, how they are obtained, their use in medicine as well as the provision of mental relaxation and well-being, i.e. aromatherapy.

J. A. von Fraunhofer
Boerne, Texas

Author's Note: *Many books and scientific articles were reviewed during the writing of this monograph. The most important of these sources are referenced as superscript numbers in the text and are listed in the Bibliography at the end of the book.*

1. INTRODUCTION

Essential oils (also known as volatile oils) are aromatic oily liquids obtained from plant or botanical materials, notably flowers, buds, seeds, leaves, twigs, bark, herbs, wood, fruits and roots. These "botanical" oils are known as essential oils because they are the "essence" of the parent plants. An estimated 3000 essential oils are known, of which 300 are commercially important in the fragrance and perfume market.[c] They can be obtained by expression, fermentation or extraction but steam distillation is the most commonly used method for commercial production (see Chapter 3 and Appendix D). Many different industries utilize essential oils to manufacture their products and, for example, attar of roses and lavender oil are important in the perfumery industry and oil of clove (eugenol) is important in dentistry. As will become clear in this book, numerous essential oils are vital in the cosmetics, food and pharmaceutical industries.

Essential oils are complex mixtures of many compounds. Chemically they are derived from terpenes and their oxygenated

---

[c] Van de Braak SAAJ, Leijten GCJJ. Essential Oils and Oleoresins: A Survey in the Netherlands and other Major Markets in the European Union. CBI, Centre for the Promotion of Imports from Developing Countries, Rotterdam. 1999.

compounds (see Appendices A and B) as well as numerous other chemical compounds in greater or lesser amounts, depending upon the individual oil. Each and every constituent contributes to the aroma or smell of the essential oil as well as to the beneficial (or adverse) effects on the body.

Looking into the availability of essential oils, I was staggered at the retail cost of what appeared to be simple, natural substances extracted from plants. For example, there is nootkatone, a citrus molecule extracted from grapefruit. Commercially, nootkatone costs about $2000 per pound and it requires about 400,000 lb. (200 tons) of grapefruit to produce 1 lb. (450 grams). of nootkatone. That is a whole lot of fruit to produce about 1 pint of fluid. As with nootkatone, a large amount of plant material is required to produce enough essential oil to fill even a small bottle. An example of this is that 22 lb. (10 kg) of rose petals must be distilled to produce just 5 ml of rose oil. When one considers that a rose petal probably weighs less than ½ g (0.018 oz.), then about 20,000 petals are needed for just 5 ml or 1 teaspoon of oil.

It is obvious that getting these essential oils from plants not only requires a lot of plant material but is both quite complex and expensive, and requires skill to achieve efficient extraction. Commercial production of pure essential oils is crucial to the flavor and fragrance industries and as mentioned above, because the processing requires specialized equipment, organically grown plants, operating skill and precise extraction procedures, they are costly. Unfortunately, this can be an open invitation for some manufacturers to adulterate essential oils to both lower costs and increase profits by incorporating synthetic ingredients into what should be wholly natural products. Interestingly, despite their economic, biological and pharmacological importance, relatively little is known about essential oils and even standard organic chemistry textbooks barely mention them.

In the preface, I mentioned that I have previously written a short monograph entitled *Vitamins, Minerals and Spices* in which I discussed these compounds and natural products that are vital to human health and gastronomy. Although I did not delve into essential oils *per se,* it is fairly obvious that these food flavorants, i.e. spices, relied on their essential oil content to confer flavor and aroma on food.

We have all experienced the evocative effects of food odors. The smell of grilled meat brings back memories of warm summer evenings in the back yard and family get-togethers around the grill. The delicious aroma of roast turkey evokes thoughts of past Thanksgiving and Christmas dinners and very little can rival the welcoming smell of baked apple or other fruit pie when one gets home after a hard day's work or even from a shopping trip on a cold winter day. Just walking into an Italian restaurant with all the delicious smells of garlic, oregano and other spices immediately stir the digestive juices. The smell of curry and many other Oriental and Far Eastern spices enhance the taste and the anticipation of eating so many different cuisines that there can almost be a sensory overload on entering these restaurants. In other words, the aromas produced by essential oils extracted from spices through cooking have an immediate and pleasing effect on the mind and body.

Given the evocative effects of liberated essential oils from plants, it is unsurprising that there is a major and steadily growing interest in the mental and physical health benefits of pleasing and satisfying scents – what is known as aromatherapy. In addition to aromatherapy, there are growing numbers of products based on essential oils that provide numerous overall mental and physical health benefits for their users.

The word *oil* is a generic term for a viscous, water-immiscible fluid. Oils have three principal sources, namely those obtained from the refining of petrochemicals, those from animal products (e.g. lard and tallow) and, thirdly, botanical or plant-based fluids. Only botanical oils are considered here although a clear distinction must be made between what are known as vegetable (culinary) oils,

Appendix B, and essential oils (EOs). Although the latter are derived from plants, as discussed below, they are obtained in a completely different manner to those used for the far more common vegetable oils and have markedly different chemical compositions, characteristics and uses. In common parlance, an *essential oil* contains the "essence" of the plant's fragrance or aroma, i.e., the characteristic smell and taste of the plant from which it is derived.

Vegetable oils are primarily used for culinary purposes whereas EOs are widely used as fragrances in cosmetics, notably perfumes, soaps and skin cremes, in pharmaceuticals, in household cleansers, and as food additives, notably for enhancing and/or modifying flavor. Essential oils also are central to aromatherapy, the practice of using essential oils to enhance feelings of psychological and physical well-being in patients, as well as in massage therapy. It follows that whereas essential oils are not *essential to life,* they are almost ubiquitous in modern living and make a major contribution to wellness and the enjoyment of life.

Finally, it is important to introduce the word *organic* which refers to foods farmed using practices that foster or promote recycling of resources and help conserve, sustain and promote ecological balance and biodiversity. Thus, in theory, organic foods are grown in the absence or limited use of pesticides, herbicides and artificial fertilizers. Further, organic foods should not have been treated with or contain synthetic food additives and have not been exposed to solvents or irradiation. Organic farming of animals and poultry implies that the same restrictions were imposed when they were raised and that they were not treated with antibiotics or exposed to radiation or pesticides in their food. Unfortunately, agrochemicals, notably pesticides, are dangerous and they are responsible for about 200,000 deaths every year with most of these fatalities occurring in developing countries.[d] Consequently, advisers

---

[d] Maria Burke. Pesticide use 'threatens human rights', UN advisers claim. Chemistry World (2017) 14(4) page 11.

have suggested to the UN Human Rights Council that pesticide use is endangering basic human rights to food and health. Further, environmental activists and Sen. Tom Udall (D-NM) are pushing legislation for the EPA (Environmental Protection Agency) to ban the use of the pesticide chlorpyrifos on food crops. This is because the organophosphate is neurotoxic and has been linked to developmental problems in children.[e] It is for these reasons that responsible producers of essential oils insist on organic farming of plants grown to make their products.

---

[e] Britt Erickson. Chemical and Engineering News (2017) 95 (31): p. 19.

J. A. von FRAUNHOFER

2. ESSENTIAL OILS

Essential oils (EOs) are concentrated hydrophobic (water-repelling) organic liquids that contain a variety of volatile aromatic compounds derived from plants. Consequently, EOs are also known as volatile oils, ethereal oils or more simply as the oils of the plants from which they were extracted. Essential oils may be inhaled as in aromatherapy (Chapter 5), taken by mouth (Chapters 4 and 8), or applied to the skin topically or by way of massage therapy (Chapters 6 and 7). They may also be applied to clothing so that body heat will release the vapor. It is important, however, to stress that essential oils are very potent and, as discussed in this book, they are highly bioactive. Consequently, they should be kept out of the hands of children[f] and caution must be exercised when essential oils are applied to the skin of babies and the very young.

Essential oils have been used by man for millennia for a variety of personal and, latterly, industrial applications. The largest use of essential oils, over 90%, is for fragrances and cosmetics. Other important applications of essential oils include personal use, aromatherapy and food flavoring. There are a great many books, reviews and articles written on essential oils (EOs) but their historic

---

[f] T. Nguyen: Unintended dietary supplement exposure on the rise. Chemical and Engineering use (2017) 95(31) p. 19

and ongoing use in medicine and human health has received less attention in the popular and scientific literature. This book will discuss the use of essential oils in these fields, which is often referred to as alternative or complementary medicine.

Essential oils are made up of a large array of chemical components, the major ones include terpenes, esters, aldehydes, ketones, phenols and oxides (see Appendix B). These compounds are volatile and contribute to the characteristic aromas (odors) of the oils. The many types of essential oils contain varying amounts of each of these compounds and the particular combinations of the many components confer the particular fragrance (and therapeutic characteristics) of each individual oil. This variability within different varieties of the same species of a plant, e.g. lavender, can be seen in Table 2.1.[1]

Table 2.1 Components (%) of the lavender plant[1]

Component	English lavender (*Lavandula angustifolia*)	Bastard lavender (*Lavandula x hybrid*)
Alcohols	30-58	31-60
Esters	26-52	32-55
Monoterpenes	7-24	7-24
Sesquiterpenes	3-9	4-10
Aldehydes	2-5	
Oxides	2-4	2-10
Coumarins	1-4	0-2
Ketones	1-3	5-11

These differences in the chemical compositions of the same plant species are known as chemotypes. Chemotyping can arise from different varieties of the same species, see Table 2.1, or other influences such as location, climate, soil quality and even the method of harvesting.[2] The marked effect of location, climate, ground water quality and mineral content, soil quality and so forth on the characteristics of plant-derived products has been recognized for centuries by a great many biotechnology industries, including olive oil, wine making, beer production, distilled liquors and even tobacco to name but a few examples. Most consumers can instantly tell the difference, for example, between olive oil from Italy, Spain, Greece and Turkey, and it is a matter of pride for wine aficionados to be able to distinguish between varietal wines produced from grapes gathered from different locations and even from different sides of the same valley where the grapes are grown. It follows, therefore, that the properties and characteristics of nominally the same essential oils will be modified when different source materials are compounded or mixed together to produce those oils.

Important components of essential oils are terpenes and terpenoids (see Appendix A) and these are thought to be the major contributors to the aromas (and characteristics) of EOs. Chemical synthesis of terpenes and terpenoids is very difficult because of their complex structures. Despite the difficulties, efforts to synthesize terpenes and terpenoids are ongoing because plants are seasonal crops that only produce small amounts of terpenes. Consequently, production of *100% pure* essential oils by extraction from their parent plants is technologically difficult, time-consuming and expensive, and is limited by crop availability. Recent research work however, has shown that it is possible to produce some essential oils by fermentation and then electrochemical oxidation of far cheaper source materials, providing substantial savings in both plant materials as well as in many other economic factors.[3,4] This recent R&D work together with many other research efforts in chemistry have increased the availability of synthetic variations and derivatives of natural terpenes and terpenoids. These developments have markedly broadened the variety of aromas used in perfumery and other applications.

Returning to question of extracting essential oils from plants, as stated previously, EOs derived from plants are not available year-round because so many of the source plants have only one growing season per year. Consequently, many suppliers of EOs circumvent this problem by using a diversity of native and foreign plant sources for their products. In other words, the source plants may be grown in the United States and in other countries to ensure a continuous supply of material. However, the quality and characteristics of EOs can be markedly affected by the soil in which the plants are grown as well as by climactic factors and the quality of the groundwater hydrating the soil. In fact, the terpene/terpenoid profile of virtually every essential oil source plant grown in one location will be different from that grown in another part of the country or overseas. This will obviously affect the characteristics, aroma and every other property of the extracted essential oil.

It should also be mentioned that many outsourced plants used for essential oil production may not be wholly *organic*. In particular, such plants may be grown using fertilizers and be exposed to toxic herbicides and pesticides. As a result, it is possible that traces of these agents are present in the so-called pure essential oils and, in the long-term, may represent a health hazard to consumers, as mentioned in Chapter 1.

3. ESSENTIAL OIL EXTRACTION

Expression or cold pressing is a method that has been used since antiquity to squeeze the juice from the seeds and sometimes the leaves of the source plants. Expression is the way the important culinary oils like olive oil, coconut oil and palm oil are produced as are fruit juices like apple, grape, orange, lime, grapefruit and lemon juice and many others. Further, lemon, lime and orange oils also are obtained by cold pressing the corresponding citrus rinds.

In contrast to production of vegetable and citrus oils as well as fruit juices, extraction of essential oils is technologically far more challenging, and is complicated by the fact that each plant contains very little essential oil, as mentioned above. There are several different approaches to extracting essential oils from botanicals; some are time-honored and others take advantage of technological advances.

<u>Enfleurage</u>
Enfleurage is one of the oldest methods of extracting and preserving the fragrances from flowering plants (botanicals) and has been a traditional method for extracting essential oils from the seeds, petals and even whole flowers of the source plant In Europe for centuries. Enfleurage was probably the method of obtaining essential oils used back in Biblical times and perhaps earlier.

Although inefficient and costly in terms of manpower, until comparatively recently enfleurage was the only method of extracting fragrant compounds from delicate flowers which might otherwise be denatured (destroyed) in the high temperatures used in distillation (see later). Now, more efficient extraction techniques such as solvent extraction and supercritical fluid extraction using a liquified gas such as carbon dioxide (CO_2) are used for delicate botanicals such as jasmine and tuberose. Nevertheless, enfleurage apparently is still used in rural areas in various parts of the world. Enfleurage is also often referred to as maceration, the scientific term for the softening of a solid by soaking so that the internal fibers separate and the delicate or highly volatile herbal essence can be leached out.

The traditional approach to fragrance extraction is known as *hot enfleurage* and involves melting solidified fats in a pot into which the botanicals are stirred. When all fragrance has been leached out from the flowers, the spent flowers are strained off and are replaced with fresh material with the process being repeated until the fat is saturated with fragrance.

The *cold enfleurage* process apparently was developed in Southern France during the 18th century for producing high-grade essential oil concentrates. In this process, a large framed plate of glass, known as a "chassis", is smeared with a layer of rendered and clarified animal fat, usually tallow or lard[g], and allowed to set. Then the botanical matter, usually flower petals but might also be whole flowers, is placed on the fat so that its scent can diffuse into the fat over 1-3 days but sometimes over a period of weeks. This process is then repeated by replacing spent botanicals with fresh ones until the fat has reached the required degree of fragrance saturation.

In both methods, the final product, fat saturated with fragrance, is known as "enfleurage pomade" or scented ointment. The pomade may either be sold as is or it can be soaked in alcohol

---

[g] Two rendered and clarified animal fats, lard and tallow, are used in enfleurage. Lard is fat from the abdomen of a pig whereas tallow comes from beef or mutton. They are rendered by slow heating with a small amount of water and then straining off the clarified fat which solidifies at room temperature.

(ethanol) to leach out the aroma compounds. After separating out any residual fat, the alcohol is allowed to evaporate off, leaving behind the "absolute" botanical, that is, *the essential oil.* Spent fat, which still retains a fair amount of fragrance, could be used to produce scented soap.

Distillation

Nowadays, the commonest commercial method of obtaining essential oils is by distillation. In this process, the source material is heated in a closed container, known as a still, to drive off the desired compound (the essential oil) from the source plant matter (usually seeds or flowers) and the liberated gaseous material is then passed from the still into an externally cooled tube where the vapor cools and condenses into a liquid to be collected in a suitable container. Classically, this is how alcoholic beverages (liquors) such as whisky, gin, rum and vodka are produced. Because the extraction procedure involves heat, there must be careful control of the distillation process to ensure that the source plants and the extracted essential oil are not damaged by the applied heat. Further, the distillation equipment must be non-reactive, e.g. fabricated from stainless steel or other non-corrodible material, to avoid contamination of the product.

Steam distillation, which is often referred to as hydrodistillation, is used to separate heat-sensitive components. It involves passing steam into the mixture or the plant matter, causing heating of the mixture and some of it to vaporize. This vapor is cooled and condensed into two liquid fractions. Sometimes the fractions are collected separately or, because they have different densities, they separate on their own. In common with vacuum distillation (see below), steam distillation is a method of achieving distillation at temperatures lower than the normal boiling point of the component to be separated. Steam distillation often is used when the component to be distilled is immiscible (incapable of mixing) with, and chemically unreactive, with water. This separation effect occurs when flowers (botanicals) are steam distilled and the distillation products are the essential oil and a water-based (aqueous) distillate.

Vacuum distillation is used to separate components in a mixture when the components have high boiling points. Lowering the pressure within the still also lowers boiling points. In most other respects, vacuum or reduced pressure distillation is essentially the same as other (simple) distillation methods. Vacuum distillation is particularly useful when the normal boiling point of a compound is greater than its decomposition temperature, i.e., the compound to be separated will be damaged or decomposed by the temperature of steam, boiling water or the heat required to volatilize it in simple or steam distillation. These are important considerations in petrochemical processing and in the extraction of certain essential oils. Whereas this methodology does have a somewhat higher operating cost, there is a lower capital cost for the construction of the distillation column. Further, because the temperatures involved in vacuum distillation are lower, there is a reduced risk of product degradation, an important factor in the petrochemical industry, but the overall process improves separation because of greater capacity, higher yields and superior product purity.

Distillation processes as well as the history of distillation are covered in greater detail in Appendix D.

Solvent extraction

Liquid or solvent extraction is another process for obtaining essential oils. In this, the source plant material is digested or treated with a solvent to dissolve out the essential oil. Such solvents include alcohol, paraffin or hexane as well as absolute oil, the latter being usually a mixture of essential oils previously extracted from plants by mineral solvents like the organic chemical hexane. Following the initial extraction process, the essential oil is separated from the carrier (the solvent or absolute oil) in a secondary operation, typically allowing the solvent to evaporate off. In many respects, solvent extraction is similar to the maceration process in enfleurage.

Inevitably with this extraction method, some solvent residues may be present in the derived essential oil. Because of this, however, oils produced with the aid of chemical solvents may not be regarded as true essential oils, because the solvent residues can alter the purity of the oils themselves, result in adulteration of the fragrance and possibly cause skin irritation.

Other extraction methods

A more modern solvent extraction method for essential oils takes advantage of the ability of liquid carbon dioxide (CO_2) to dissolve out the oil from the botanical (plant) source without heat. Although liquid CO_2 extraction may have a higher cost than the more traditional distillation and solvent methods and requires specialized equipment, it does have the advantage of not leaving solvent residue in the essential oil. This approach is often used for vanilla oil extraction.

In recent years, there has been increasing interest in solvent-free microwave extraction (SFME), also known as microwave "dry" distillation or microwave accelerated distillation (MAD).[5,6,7] This extraction technique is a combination of microwave heating and dry distillation which is performed at normal or atmospheric pressure without requiring any solvent or water. Not only is this approach considered to be "green", data indicates that extraction is faster and more efficient than the traditional methods. While SFME/MAD has obvious advantages for small scale extractions, it is debatable whether this methodology could readily be scaled up for bulk extraction of essential oils. There is also ongoing interest in using other technologies for essential oil extraction, including laser heating of the plant material.

Commercial Production

As has already been discussed, spices, vegetable oils and essential oils are central to modern living and their supply and demand have spawned numerous large and important industries that manufacture and market culinary spices, cosmetics, food flavorings, fragrances and a host of other products. Even a cursory review of the production, packaging and marketing of essential oils indicates that EOs are big business, as shown by the list of many retail suppliers of essential oils, Table 3.1, and there appear to be just as many National and International wholesale suppliers of these important products. The commercial importance of essential oils and their associated industries can lead to the misperception that this important field is a modern phenomenon. In fact, essential oils, perfumes and spices have been around since the dawn of civilization, Appendix C.

The yields of essential oils from plants are low because their average essential oil content is only 1-3% although the resins of Frankincense and Myrrh are typically much higher at 3-9%. Thus, in most cases, a ton or more of flowers may be required to produce 0.5 kg (1 lb.) of essential oil and about 400,000 kg (nearly 1 ton) of grapefruits, for example, is needed to produce 1 kg (2.2 lb.) of nootkatone, which is present in grapefruit and certain cedar trees. Whereas the sesquiterpene nootkatone, a compound found in grapefruit, is not an essential oil itself, it is a significant component of many essential oils.

This limited yield of essential oils, botanical seasonality and the economic and technological demands of processing accounts for the cost of essential oils, their relative scarcity and, sometimes, only intermittent availability. A corollary to this is that it is highly unlikely that "pure" essential oils costing only a few dollars and found in many supermarkets, drug stores and on line are pure products. It may also be questionable whether the source plants were organically grown or derived from a single plant source.

Table 3.1. Commercial suppliers of Essential Oils

Aromaland

ArtNaturals

Citrus and Allied Essences

doTERRA

Eden's Garden

Essential Oil Company

Fleurchem Inc.

Gurunanda

Lebermuth Company

Liberty Natural Products

Miracle Essential Oils

New Directions Aromatics

NHR Organic Oils

Now Solutions

Organic Infusions

Plant Therapy Essential Oils

Rocky Mountain Oils

Wellington Fragrance Company

Young Living

J. A. von FRAUNHOFER

4. ESSENTIAL OILS IN THE 21ST CENTURY

Many therapeutic approaches have been used by man for hundreds and often thousands of years to treat a wide variety of human ailments and both mental and physical conditions, Table 4.1. The scientific term for herbal-based traditional medical practices that use plant materials for both preventive and therapeutic is phytomedicine. Even in the 21st Century, according to the WHO, up to 80% of the population in some Asian and African countries relies on traditional medicine for their primary health care needs.[8] Despite their widespread appeal and claimed effectiveness, when many of these traditional or folk remedies and therapies are used outside of their native cultures, they are commonly referred to as *complementary therapy* or *alternative medicine*. Further, complementary or alternative medicine (CAM) therapies are generally not recognized by Government agencies and organized medicine in developed countries. Nevertheless, as discussed later, topical treatment with essential oils has shown possible value for fungal infections and hair loss. Further, oral use of essential oils may also treat various digestive and respiratory problems.

Many suppliers of essential oils advance a variety of health-related claims for essential oils, Table 4.2, and many claims are made regarding the antibacterial properties of certain EOs as well as for a variety of herbs and spices.[9] However, none of these claims have been evaluated or are approved by the FDA and the use of essential oils for medicinal purposes should not replace proper medical treatment when indicated or displace personal judgment in treating any pathological condition. Of equal importance is that none of these health benefit claims should be understood to diagnose, treat, cure or prevent any disease.

Table 4.1. Traditional (folk) medicine and alternate (complementary) therapies

Acupuncture	Islamic medicine
Ancient Persian medicine	Massage therapy
Aromatherapy	Muti Ifa
Ayurvedic medicine	Naturopathic medicine
Chiropractic	Shamanism
Essential oil therapy	Siddha medicine
Ethnomedicine	Traditional African Medicine
Folk medicine	Traditional Chinese medicine
Herbalism	Traditional Korean medicine
Holistic medicine	Unani
Homeopathy	Veganism

Table 4.2. Essential Oils and Their Claimed Health Benefits

Note: Many essential oils, and their parent plants and ground-up seeds, have been used for millennia in cooking. This use is based on their well-established effects on the taste of food and on mood and emotions, as well as for their purported beneficial effects on health. These oils used for culinary purposes are marked with an asterisk (*).

Essential Oil	Claimed Health Benefit or Application
Basil*	Mental alertness, sore muscles/joints, menstruation pain, insect bites
Bergamot*	Skin purifying, emotional support
Birch	Muscles and joint health, skin blemishes, mood elevation
Black pepper*	Antioxidant, healthy circulation, food flavoring

Cardamom*	Digestion, respiratory health, food flavoring
Cassia	Healthy cell function, digestion, mood enhancement
Cedarwood	Skin health, emotional support, insect repellant
Chamomile*	Calming effect, immune system health
Cilantro*	Antioxidant, digestive aid, cleansing, skin health
Cinnamon	Metabolic function, oral health, cleaning
Clary sage	Hormonal balance, tension relief, emotional support, emolient for rashes, antibacterial agent.
Clove*	Cardiovascular health, dentistry, immune system, food flavoring
Coriander*	Digestion aid, skin health, sore joints and muscles
Cumin*	Digestive health, body system purification, food flavoring
Cypress	Muscle relaxant, energy booster, skin health
Dill*	Digestive support, emotional support, food flavoring
Douglas Fir	Respiratory health, skin health
Eucalyptus	Respiration support, skin health, cleansing
Fennel*	Digestive aid, metabolic support, circulatory aid
Frankincense	Cellular health, skin purifier, emotional support
Geranium	Healthy skin and hair, emotional support, insect repellant
Ginger*	Digestive support, emotional support, food flavoring, antioxidant
Grapefruit*	Cleansing, skin health, metabolic health, mental acuity
Helichrysum	Skin health, metabolic support
Jasmine	Skin health, balanced mood
Juniper berry*	Kidney/urinary function, skin appearance, stress relief, food flavoring

Lavender	Wide applicability, skin health, emotional support, food flavoring, antiseptic
Lemon*	Energy support, digestive and respiratory health, cleaning
Lemongrass*	Digestive health, muscle/joint pain, skin health, insect repellant
Lime*	Detoxification, healthy immune function, energy stimulant
Marjoram*	Emotional support, muscle relaxant, cardiovascular function
Melissa (Lemon balm)	Immune system support, stress relief
Myrrh	Skin health, emotional support, antibacterial action
Orange*	Emotional balance, overall health, antioxidant, food flavoring
Oregano*	Immune/digestion/respiratory system health, food flavoring
Patchouli	Skin health/complexion, emotional support
Peppermint*	Digestive/respiratory system support, energy enhancement, food flavoring
Rose	Skin health, emotional balance, perfumery
Rosemary*	Digestive aid, respiratory support, hair/scalp health, food flavoring
Sage (Salvia)*	Mood enhancement
Sandalwood	Skin health, emotional support, perfume
Spearmint*	Digestive health, oral health, food flavoring
Tangerine*	Immune system support, food flavoring
Tea Tree (Melaleuca)	Immune system support, skin health, antiseptic
Thyme*	Immune system support, food flavoring, insect repellent
Vanilla	Promotes skin and hair health, relieves muscle pain and cramps, hormonal balancing
Vetiver	Immune system support, emotional support
White fir	Supports and treats muscle and joint pain, emotional support

Wild Orange	Emotional balance, overall health, cleansing/purifying, antioxidants
Wintergreen*	Muscle/joint pain, skin health, emotional support, scent
Ylang Ylang	Skin, scalp and hair health, emotional support

The systemic health effects of essential oils may be questionable although many of the above oils have been certified as GRAS (Generally Recognized as Safe) by the FDA for oral consumption, see Chapter 6. The topical use of certain essential oils to promote wound healing and prevent infection has been advocated for millennia, and this contention is supported modern research studies, see Chapters 6 and 8. There is also a growing scientific literature on the therapeutic value of certain essential oils in the treatment of a variety of conditions. Peppermint oil alone and in combination with caraway oil, for example, is reported to be effective for a variety of gastric problems.[10,11,12,13,14]

Finally, the scientific literature indicates that sesquiterpenoids, and specifically sesquiterpene lactones, i.e. essential oils, extracted from the Asteraceae family (e.g., asters, daisies and sunflowers) may play an important role in human health due to their potential for the treatment of cardiovascular disease and cancer.[15] This may be as part of the diet and as pharmaceutical agents. Interestingly, there is also increasing scientific evidence that certain essential oils are effective in cancer prevention and treatment.[8,16,17,18,19,20,21,22,23,24,25]

Scientific evidence clearly shows that medicinal plants and probiotics are beneficial to health through their antimicrobial activity against antibiotic-resistant enteric pathogens.[26,27] Probiotics are themselves enteric microorganisms that have no parasitic effect on man (or animals) and have been an integral part of daily food for centuries.[28,29,30,31] The widespread use of probiotics is due, at least in part, because of their beneficial effect on the gut by inhibiting or retarding the growth of microorganisms. Many essential oils are believed to kill bacteria, i.e. are bactericidal (see Chapter 8), and there is growing interest in combining medicinal plant extracts and probiotics to take advantage of their complementary antimicrobial effects with virtually no side effects. In other words, there is a synergism between the essential oil and probiotics that exerts a greater effect than that found when using them alone.

5. AROMATHERAPY

Odors, namely smells, scents and aromas, have an evocative, almost subliminal effect on the mind. As any realtor will tell you, the way to enhance the appeal of a home is to bake an apple pie or chocolate chip cookies prior to an open house or showing the place to a prospective buyer. Likewise, the smell of meat or onions cooking on a grill have an almost Pavlovian effect on the salivary glands, even when the grill can be out of sight.

The calming effects of perfumes and their effect on other human emotions have been recognized since Biblical times but the therapeutic application of essential oils was only recognized as a separate discipline in the early 1900s.[32,33,34] Interestingly, the first major figures in modern aromatherapy, the French chemist and perfumer René-Maurice Gattefossé, and his fellow countryman and aromatherapist, the physician Jean Valnet. These men were the first to document the use of essential oils for medical purposes, notably the treatment of skin infections and wounds (see Chapter 8).[1,2,3] Although Gattefossé was both a chemist and perfumer, when he coined the term *aromatherapie* (French for aromatherapy) in 1920s and 1930s, he was referring to the treatment of disease and injury using aromatic essential oils rather than the modern use of the term for the beneficial effects of inhaling EOs.

The early reports of the beneficial effects of aromas on the mind and body have been expanded upon by numerous workers in the field. Scientific studies using electroencephalogram (EEC) patterns and functional imaging techniques have shown that odors and aromas can produce specific effects on human neuropsychological and autonomic function and can have such emotional effects as influencing mood, perceived health, and arousal.[35] Such studies consistently show that odors can produce specific effects on human neuropsychological and autonomic function; in other words, aromas can influence mood, perceived health and even arousal, common effects induced by perfumes. The indications are that the effect of essential oils on brainwaves and behavior modification appears most probably transmitted through the brain via the olfactory system.[36]

Aromatherapy is a form of herbal medicine that uses essential oils, i.e., the natural oils extracted from flowers, bark, stems, leaves, roots or other plant parts to enhance the quality of life by improving the psychological, spiritual and physical well-being of the patient or user.[37,38,39] Thus, aromatherapy improves the quality of life (QOL). Although considered to be yet another form of alternative medicine, aromatherapy is used or is claimed to be useful for a vast array of symptoms and conditions. Aromatherapy, for example, is increasingly used for a variety of applications, including mood enhancement, i.e., stress relief and reduction of anxiety and depression, to limit pain and to improve cognitive function.[40,41,42] Thus, most scientific studies of aromatherapy are directed at its psychological effects, notably stress relief and anxiolytic action. It should be noted, however, that such noted advocates of antibacterial activity of essential oils, namely Gattefossé and Valnet (see Chapter 8), referred to this use as "aromatherapy". Other workers have used a similar nomenclature in reporting their research studies with essential oils. In the context of this book, "aromatherapy" refers only to inhalation effects of aerially diffused essential oils, as discussed below.

Commonly in aromatherapy, essential oils are evaporated into the air by means of a humidifier or diffuser although, as indicated in Chapter 4 and later in Chapters 6 and 7, essential oils may also be applied directly to the skin or onto clothing so that they release their odor (aroma) immediately to the patient. A popular and well-established application of this principle is Vicks VapoRub, a gel based on a combination of the essential oils of peppermint, eucalyptus, and camphor. This classic aromatic ointment is a topical cough medicine with medicated vapors that works quickly for children and adults to relieve cough and nasal congestion. In this context, a book on aromatherapy in children suggests remedies for treating pertussis (whooping cough) and as a topical treatment for skin-related conditions such as acne.[43]

The principal methods of utilizing aromatherapy are:
- Arial diffusion for environmental fragrancing and purification;[44]
- Direct inhalation for respiratory disinfection, decongestion and stimulation   of expectoration as well as psychological effects; and
- Topical application in massaging, bathing, compresses and skin care.

Essential oils recommended for aromatherapy are indicated in Table 5.1 at the end of this chapter. Certain essential oil producers also formulate oil blends to achieve specific aromatherapy effects. Most of these pure oils and blends can be applied directly, i.e. topically, to the skin although the packaging should be checked to determine whether the oil or blend should be diluted with a carrier oil to avoid skin irritation. This is important for users with sensitive skins or a history of eczema or dermatitis.

The basis for aromatherapy is that the inhaled vaporized matter and aroma from the essential oils is perceived to stimulate brain function, a perception supported by scientific evidence.[4] Further, because essential oils also can be absorbed through the skin, topical application of EOs is believed to promote whole-body healing because they are transported throughout the body by means of the bloodstream.[45] Several essential oils, including lavender, rose, orange, bergamot, lemon, sandalwood, salvia, and chamomile, are widely believed to be effective anxiolytic (anxiety-reducing) agents.

Although aromatherapy is increasingly popular and has made its way into the offices of health care providers and into spas and homes, there are few clear indications for its therapeutic use. In fact, it is very difficult to scientifically evaluate the clinical effectiveness of inhaled essential oils because patients in a clinical trial are immediately aware that they are inhaling an aromatic substance. Because the trial participants can smell the aroma, they are likely to expect a beneficial effect and will respond affirmatively when asked about their reactions by the testing scientists regardless of whether or not the anticipated benefits really exist. Nevertheless, the belief of the majority of health care workers using aromatherapy as well as the findings of the limited number of controlled scientific studies all indicate that aromatherapy can have a beneficial effect in relieving anxiety and depression as well as reducing post-operative nausea and vomiting.[4,6,7,9] Clinical trials continue world-wide to validate or dismiss the health benefit claims of aromatherapy but the consensus is that aromatherapy can be effective in many situations. An example of the beneficial effects of aromatherapy is in the treatment of individuals in emotional distress. Patients are often treated with psychotherapeutic agents but it is reported that a safe and effective adjunct for the prevention and treatment of emotional distress is aromatherapy.[46]

Aromatherapy products do not need approval by the FDA and different aromatherapists use various combinations of oils, and methods of application, to treat specific conditions. Differences in oil combinations and methods of use are practitioner-dependent although some approaches are more widely accepted than others throughout the aromatherapy community.

Although training and certification in aromatherapy for lay (non-medical) practitioners is available at several schools throughout the United States and in many other countries, there is no professional standardization in the United States, and no license is required to practice aromatherapy in the USA. As a result, there is little consistency between practitioners in the treatments used for specific illnesses or conditions. One result of this lack of standardization is that there tends to be inconsistency in research studies on the effects of aromatherapy. In part, this is because tradition, anecdotal evidence and the prior experience of the practitioner determine the essential oil selection. Consequently, the choice of oils by researchers can often be quite arbitrary when studying the same applications.

This situation is now changing, with specific courses being available for healthcare professionals and caregivers wanting to become aromatherapist. These courses often satisfy continuing medical education contact hour requirements for healthcare professionals and many also include a research component and provide information on evaluating aromatherapy outcomes. As a result, the landscape of aromatherapy is changing and improving.

At least two governing bodies, The National Association for Holistic Aromatherapy and The Alliance of International Aromatherapists, are working to establish national educational standards and to standardize aromatherapy certification for aromatherapists. The Canadian Federation of Aromatherapists also has established standards for aromatherapy certification in Canada and has standards for safety and professional conduct. Such organizations likely exist in many other countries. It should also be mentioned that whereas aromatherapy in the USA is generally limited to inhalation or topical application, aromatherapists in France and Germany often administer essential oils orally or internally.

Finally, although many research studies on aromatherapy have been conducted with synthetic oils, most aromatherapists believe that synthetic fragrances are inferior to pure essential oils because they lack "natural or vital energy". This contention has been challenged by psychologists and biochemists working in this field.[47]

Table 5.1 Aromatherapy Oils

Although most essential oils can be used in diffusers for aromatherapy, the following are the ones advocated for their calming or relaxation properties (*), for spiritual uplifting and inspiration (#), for energizing effects (^) or to improve concentration (%). The usual application rate is 8-12 drops of essential oil to ½ cup (4 oz.) of distilled water in a diffuser.

Note that the comments made here have not been evaluated by the Food and Drug Administration (FDA) and none of these products are intended to diagnose, treat, cure or prevent any disease.

Angelica*	Grapefruit^	Palmarosa*
Basil*	Helichrysum%	Palo Santo#
Bergamot*#	Hinoki#	Patchouli*
Black pepper^	Hong Kuai#%	Peppermint*
Cardamom#	Hyssop%	Petitgrain^
Carrot seed*	Idaho balsam fir*	Pine*
Cedarwood*	Idaho blue spruce*	Ravintsara#
Celery seed*		Rose*#
Cinnamon bark^	Jade lemon^	Rosemary#
Cistus*#	Jasmine*	Royal Hawaiian sandalwood#%
Clary sage*	Juniper*	Sacred frankincense#%
Coriander*#	Laurus Nobilis^	
Cypress*	Ledum^	Sage*%
Dill*	Lemon myrtle^	Spearmint*#
Eucalyptus blue*^	Lime^	Tangerine^

Eucalyptus Radiata^	Mastrante*	Taragon*
Fennel#	Melissa#^	Thyme%
Frankincense*#	Myrrh#	Valerian*
Galbanum^	Myrtle^	Vetiver*
Geranium*#	Neroli^	Wintergreen#%
German chamomile*	Northern Lights black spruce#%	Xiang Mao#
Ginger^	Nutmeg^	Ylang Ylang*
Goldenrod*	Orange*%	

6. TOPICAL APPLICATION of ESSENTIAL OILS

The skin is the largest organ in the human body and is an essential barrier that protects the body against pathogens and prevents excessive water loss.[48,49] Other vital functions of the skin include regulation of the body temperature, insulation, permitting touch sensations such as heat sensitivity and the production of Vitamin D through the effect of sunlight.

Skin has a two-fold structure, namely the outermost layer, the epidermis, and the innermost layer, the dermis, the two being separated by a thin sheet of fibers called the basement membrane. The epidermis provides the external barrier whereas the dermis cushions the body from stresses and strains. The thickness of skin varies across the body and contains pores that allow it to breathe and permit outward passage of water (i.e. sweat) and oils through it; that is, skin is permeable. Pore size also varies across the body, being wider on the soles of the feet than elsewhere. Consequently, certain areas of the body are more permeable than others, notably the forehead and scalp, soles of the feet, the palms of the hand, the genitals, the armpits and mucous membranes.

Skin can absorb essential oils because of their small molecular size and, additionally, because they can interact with lipid molecules (tissue fats) within the skin. It is, therefore, almost intuitively obvious that applying essential oils to the skin, i.e. topical application, will have various effects on the body due to their ready absorption. Other direct and indirect topical applications include mixing essential oils in bath salts and lotions or applying them to wound dressings. The latter use, which takes advantage of antimicrobial action of EOs, is discussed in Chapter 8. A common topical use of essential oils is massage therapy (see Chapter 7).

Before continuing the discussion of the topical use of essential oils, it is worth mentioning that such noted advocates of this application of essential oils, namely Gattefossé and Valnet (see Chapter 8), referred to this practice as "aromatherapy". Other workers have used a similar nomenclature in reporting their research studies with essential oils.

Many claims are made for topical treatment using essential oils, including relief of muscle and joint pain, counteracting skin and fungal infections (see Chapter 8), treating hair loss and for various digestive and respiratory problems, and for relief of insect bites. Oral use of essential oils may treat certain conditions, notably periodontal problems and aphthous ulceration (recurrent round or oval sores inside the mouth).[50,51,52,53]

In any discussion of the topical application of essential oils, it is important to sound a note of caution. Because of their potency, users should be cautious when topically applying essential oils. The American Academy of Dermatology and other professional bodies indicate that fragrances (i.e. perfumes and cosmetics) are the leading cause of contact dermatitis (skin irritation). In fact, cutaneous (skin) sensitivity affects more than 2 million people in the USA alone and it appears that this type of sensitivity is on the rise. Since fragrances contain essential oils, caution must be exercised in their use because components within the essential oil may bind with proteins in the skin to cause the sensitizing response of allergic contact dermatitis. Further, essential oils as supplied are strong, highly concentrated fluids and some *may* cause irritation. A listing of some EOs that *may cause* irritation is given in Table 6.1. There are, however, many essential oils, notably frankincense, lavender, melaleuca (tea tree oil), melissa and sandalwood, that are generally recognized as less likely to cause sensitivity issues and often are used undiluted by adults (see below).

Caution in the topical use of essential oils is especially true for those with sensitive skin or when the EO is to be applied to young children or babies. In these cases, users are strongly advised to both dilute the EO in a carrier oil and to test the diluted oil in a small inconspicuous area of the skin to check for irritation and/or sensitivity. Not only that, essential oils should never be applied near mucous membranes such as those in or around the eyes, the nose, the ears, the vagina and anus. Likewise, essential oils, including gels such as VapRub, should never be applied within the nostrils although some practitioners advocate placing a few drops beneath the nostrils to relieve nasal congestion.

Table 6.1 Essential oils that may cause skin irritation

Basil	Eucalyptus	Pine
Bergamot	Fir Needle	Rosemary
Camphor	Ginger	Spruce
Cassia	Lemongrass	Thyme
Cinnamon	Oregano	White fir
Clary Sage	Peppermint	Wintergreen

Although many oils may be used as carriers or diluents for EOs, most practitioners recommend those listed in Table 6.2. Some essential oil producers also market vegetable oil blends specifically formulated as carriers for pure essential oils.

Table 6.2 Suitable Carrier Oils for Essential Oils

Almond oil
Aloe Vera oil
Argan oil
Fractionated coconut oil
Grape seed oil
Jojoba oil
Neem oil
Rosehip oil
Sesame seed oil
Sunflower seed oil
Vanilla oil

These "carrier" oils and vegetable oils with a high polyunsaturated fat content.[h] are more easily absorbed by the skin than thicker oils like olive oil. It should also be noted that certain producers of essential oils, e.g. Young Living, offer specialty oil mixtures that are used to dilute the highly concentrated essential oils before they are applied to individuals with sensitive skin and also for creating custom massage oils.

Essential oil dilution is often a matter of trial and error but 1 drop of EO in 1 tablespoon of carrier oil (i.e. about 0.2% dilution) is typical for babies, infants and young children whereas 2 drops of essential oil per teaspoon of carrier oil (0.75%) is more suitable for adults. In massage therapy, however, dilutions of 2-5% are more common.

The common areas for applying essential oils, and the anticipated effects, are noted in Table 6.3. The recommend method of using essential oils is to *gently* rub them into the skin.

---

[h] Fractionated coconut oil is coconut oil that has been treated to remove long-chain triglycerides to produce a thin, odorless, non-greasy liquid that is quickly absorbed by the skin; further, it does not interact with, or change the chemical composition of, the essential oil].

Table 6.3 Areas for Topical Essential Oil Application

Area	Projected Effect
Face	Skin beautification and smoothing, improved complexion
Forehead, temples and neck	Relief of tension, calming effect
Behind the ears	Relaxation, tension relief
Arms, legs and back	Muscle relaxation, easing joint stiffness and pain
Soft palate (roof of the mouth)	Relaxation, tension relief
Chest	Improved respiration, congestion relief
Abdomen	Improved digestion
Soles of the feet	Total relaxation, feeling of general wellbeing, energization, immune system support

Most massage therapists recommend applying essential oils to the bottom of the feet because there the skin is thicker, the pores are large, there are fewer nerve ending so that the oils more readily enter the blood stream. It is well known that anything applied to the sole of the feet rapidly enters the blood stream and, for example, when tincture of iodine is dabbed on the sole, it is tasted within the mouth in a matter of minutes! Obviously, the faster the EO enters the blood stream, the more rapid is the onset of the desired effect.

Interestingly, scientific studies[54,55,56] have shown that topical use of lavender and lavender-thymol reduces perineal discomfort following episiotomy[i] and promotes episiotomy healing. In fact, this use of lavender oil essence may be preferable to the skin antiseptic Betadine (Povidone-iodine) widely-used or episiotomy wound care with few or no expected side effects.

---

[i] An episiotomy is a surgical cut made at the opening of the vagina during childbirth to aid a difficult delivery and prevent rupture of tissues.

<u>Essential Oils for the Hair and Scalp</u>

Hair loss/baldness, known by the medical term alopecia, occurs with both men and women but is more common with males and known as androgenetic alopecia. When hair is lost from some or all areas of the body in spots but commonly from the scalp, the condition is known as alopecia areata.

Alopecia has many causes, including stress, poor nutrition, elevated levels of DHT (dihydrotestosterone) and scalp tissue problems such as dehydration, poor circulation, inflammation and blocked hair follicles. The psychological effects of hair loss are well-known[57,58,59] and many sufferers invest in topical hair-restorer products or hair replacement surgery in the hope of regaining full heads of hair. Although the latter is usually effective, it is relatively expensive whereas, by and large, most commercial topical hair restorative products are ineffective at best. Consequently, alopecia sufferers tend to accept the status quo or adopt palliative measures such as toupees, wigs or wearing assorted head coverings and it is not uncommon for balding men to completely shave their heads.

Proponents of essential oils and their many uses have long claimed that certain essential oils can cure or at least ameliorate alopecia by their action on the scalp and the hair. Table 6.4 indicates which essential oils are claimed to stimulate hair growth and reverse hair loss.

Table 6.4 Essential Oils for the Hair and Scalp

Essential oil	Claimed Action
Cedarwood	Stimulates the hair follicles by increasing circulation to the scalp
Chamomile	Soothes the scalp, shines and softens hair and can lighten hair color
Clary sage	Helps regulate oil production in the scalp to prevent dandruff
Lavender	Soothes the scalp, deepens hair follicle depth, thickens dermal layer

Lemongrass oil	Strengthens hair follicles, soothes itchy/irritated scalps, reduces dandruff
Peppermint	Stimulates the scalp, treats dandruff and head lice, promotes hair growth
Rosemary	Enhances hair growth, thickens hair by increasing cellular metabolism

These essential oils are usually used with a carrier such as olive, coconut or jojoba oil and, after being gently massaged into the scalp, are left in place for 1-2 hours or even overnight before being removed by shampooing.

Most trichologists dismiss such claims as anecdotal at best or simply *old wives' tales*. There is, however, a growing body of scientific literature that indicates essential oils may in fact improve scalp health and stimulate hair growth.

A recent study performed on mice[60] compared the effects of minoxidil with a 3% and 5% solution of lavender oil in jojoba oil when applied once a day, 5 times a week for 4 weeks. All three agents showed a significantly increased number of hair follicles, deepened hair follicle depth and thickened dermal layer. In other words, the results indicated that lavender oil has a marked hair growth-promoting effect.

Another recent study performed on human subjects[61] compared the effects of rosemary oil in jojoba oil with a 2% minoxidil solution in the treatment of alopecia over a 6-month period. Both groups experienced a significant increase in hair count at 3-months and at the 6-month endpoint compared with the baseline and there was no significant difference between the study groups regarding hair count either at 3 or 6 months. Of note was that no differences in the prevalence of dry hair, greasy hair and dandruff were found between the test groups at 3 and 6 months although the frequency of scalp itching was significantly higher than that at the start of the study for both test groups. Interestingly, scalp itching was more frequent with the minoxidil group compared to that with the rosemary oil group. The findings of this study confirmed a much earlier study[62] on the treatment of alopecia areata. In this study, termed *aromatherapy* by the authors, essential oils (thyme, rosemary, lavender and cedarwood) in a mixture of carrier oils (jojoba and grapeseed) were massaged daily into the scalp and compared with the effect of the carrier oils alone of alopecia areata over a 7-month period. The results showed "aromatherapy" to be a safe and effective treatment for alopecia areata and significantly more effective than treatment with the carrier oil alone.

The effect of peppermint oil on hair growth mice has also been studied, using the same type of mice as that used in the lavender oil study cited above.[63]. The effects on hair growth of topical applications of saline, jojoba oil, 3% minoxidil and 3% peppermint oil were compared over a 4-week period. The study showed that the peppermint oil treatment showed the most prominent hair growth effects, notably a significant increase in dermal thickness, follicle number, and follicle depth and there was no effect on body weight gain and food efficiency.

Natural remedies for treating dandruff are becoming increasingly popular (Table 6.4). Another recent study[64] has shown that daily use of hair tonic containing 5, 10 or 15%. lemongrass oil significantly reduced dandruff at 7 days by 33, 75 and 51% respectively and the reduction was even greater (by 52, 81 and 74% respectively) at 14-days. Interestingly, the findings indicate that a lemongrass oil content of 10% appeared to be the optimal level for effective dandruff treatment.

The studies cited here clearly indicate that essential oils show a great deal of promise for the effective treatment of hair and scalp conditions such as dandruff and alopecia (hair loss). They also indicate that anecdotal reports of the effectiveness of EOs in slowly and even reversing hair loss have a sound scientific basis

The topical application of essential oils to larger areas of the skin, notably as massage therapy, is discussed in the next chapter.

7. MASSAGE THERAPY

Massage therapy[65,66,67,67] is a venerable traditional for relieving muscle and joint pain. The practice dates back over thousands of years and references to massage have been noted in ancient writings from China, Egypt, India and Japan.

According to a recent report[j], 41.6% of adults in 2012 with a musculoskeletal pain disorder used one or more complementary or alternative medicine (CAM) health care approaches for treatment.[68] An even higher prevalence of use was seen among persons who had neck pain and problems (50.6%) and other musculoskeletal complications (46.2%). The prevalence, and popularity, of CAM therapies is not unexpected because about one quarter to one third of adults might be suffering from one or more of these disorders in any given year. Further, many forms of chronic pain are resistant to conventional medical treatment other than analgesics (pain killers). Interestingly, approximately 1% of adult CAM users utilized it to treat sinusitis (1.2%), elevated cholesterol (1.1%), asthma (1.1%), hypertension (1.0%), and/or menopause pain and discomfort (0.8%).[64-67] Included in the category of CAM therapies (see Table 4.1) is massage therapy and it is estimated that about 18 million U.S. adults and 700,000 children receive massage therapy each year, and the numbers are growing.

---

[j] National Health Statistics Report No. 98 (October 12, 2016)

People seek massage therapy for a variety of health-related issues.[64-67] These include, but are not limited to, pain relief, stress reduction and relaxation, rehabilitation of sports injuries and as a means of relieving anxiety and depression, as noted above. In general, massage therapists work on muscles and other soft tissues using long strokes as well as kneading, applying deep circular pressure movements and vibration, and often tapping. This massage technique is commonly known as Swedish massage. Sports massage utilizes Swedish massage combined with deep tissue pressure application to release chronic muscle tension, a technique primarily used for athletes. Other techniques include deep tissue massage and trigger point massage; the latter focuses on myofascial trigger points, the so-called muscle "knots" that are painful when pressed and can cause both localized pain and discomfort as well as symptoms elsewhere in the body. It also appears that many cultures have developed their own, often quite unique, approaches to massage. This approach is common in Thailand, China, Japan, India and many Middle Eastern countries to name but a few.

In massage therapy, the physical work on muscles etc. is often performed in conjunction with the application of essential oils so that patients also receive the additional benefit of aromatherapy. This combination of aromatherapy and massage therapy is often referred to as *aromatherapy massage*. The most commonly used essential oils for massage are listed in Table 7.1 although some suppliers of essential oils do compound "massage oils" and Young Living, for example, formulates and markets six different massage oils, including one for sensitive skins, that are designed for different and quite specific massage therapy procedures.

Table 7.1 Essential oils commonly used in massage therapy

Basil
Coriander
German chamomile
Ginger
Lemongrass
Marjoram
Mountain savory
Oregano
Palo Santo
Thyme
Valerian
Wintergreen

Massage therapists that combine aromatherapy with massage (i.e. aromatherapy massage) often have their own favorite essential oil combinations to achieve certain desired effects. However, coconut oil is a primary ingredient for most massage oils.

Over at least the past 30 or so years, there have been a lot of scientific studies that have attempted to evaluate, and quantify, the beneficial effects of massage therapy. Because the perceived benefits of massage therapy are individualistic and highly subjective, it is almost impossible to perform scientific studies that will provide verifiable and reproducible data or research findings that can be evaluated using statistical analysis, the "yard stick" of science. As a result, opinions and data on massage therapy and aromatherapy massage are predominantly consensus-based rather scientifically validated research findings. Nevertheless, the bulk of evidence indicates massage therapy and aromatherapy massage is beneficial in addressing and alleviating pain and other symptoms associated with many different conditions[69,70,71,72,73,74,75,76,77,78,79], as shown in Table 7.2.

Table 7.2 Conditions benefitting from massage therapy/aromatherapy massage

Muscle and joint pain
Back pain
Osteoarthritis
Mental health/relaxation
Anxiety relief
Headaches
Fibromyalgia
Infant and child care
Asthma
HIV/AIDS
Pain and nausea associated with cancer and chemotherapy

Obviously, there are many other applications of this venerable CAM technique. Despite the absence of valid evidence-based scientific data from scientific research, the overall evidence suggests that there are benefits arising from massage therapy. However, these beneficial outcomes are generally of a short-term effectiveness and repeat treatment is usually necessary and on a regular basis to maintain full and effective benefits. Further, many reports on massage therapy are conflicting and, for example, there appears to be little effectiveness with massage therapy for asthma sufferers.[75] Likewise, a critical search of the literature for clinical trials involving massage with or without aromatherapy for symptom relief in people with cancer indicated that many studies were of very low quality.[77,78] Whereas some studies suggest that massage without aromatherapy may help relieve short-term pain and anxiety in people with cancer, others indicate that aromatherapy massage may provide medium- or long-term relief for these symptoms.[77,78] Clearly, more research, preferably involving carefully controlled clinical trials, is necessary.

Despite the widespread and increasingly popular use of massage therapy and aromatherapy massage for treating conditions as varied as childhood autism, asthma, HIV/AIDS and cancer pain alleviation, just how these CAM therapies work is unknown. One theory is that the stimulation provided by massage helps block or interfere with pain signals sent to the brain. This is known by various names but commonly as the *gate control theory* and implies that there is a limited amount of sensory input to the brain and anything that constricts or blocks neural pathways will provide pain relief. Other people have suggested that massage and aromatherapy massage stimulate the release of chemicals known as neurotransmitters in the body, notably endorphins and serotonin. Endorphins are morphine-like chemicals produced by the body which help reduce pain sensations while triggering positive feelings. In simple terms, endorphins often are called the "feel-good" chemicals in the brain and are the body's natural painkillers. Serotonin is a natural mood stabilizer and is involved in many body processes, including wound healing, sleep, eating and digestion as well as helping diminish depression and regulating anxiety. Based on the activities of these neurotransmitters in the brain and throughout the body, their release through massage therapy and aromatherapy massage should be effective in relieving pain and many other conditions.

Many health care providers receive training in massage therapy and aromatherapy massage, notably physical therapists, osteopaths and chiropractors. In addition, there are also about 1,500 or more massage training programs and massage therapy schools in the United States. The majority of these training programs are approved by a state licensing board and/or by independent agencies such as the Commission on Massage Therapy Accreditation (COMTA). Licensed/certified massage therapists usually have received at least 500 hours of training, were required to pass national examinations and satisfy specific continuing education (CE) requirements on an annual or bi-annual basis. As a result, when performed by a properly trained therapist and if appropriate cautions are followed, massage therapy should have few serious risks or adverse side-effects. However, even with the most skilled practitioner, there can be temporary side-effects like pain, discomfort, bruising or swelling. Again, although uncommon, aromatherapy massage can be associated with skin sensitivity or even allergic reactions to the massage oils being used.

Regardless of the numerous anecdotal reports of the benefits of massage therapy and aromatherapy massage, and their widespread and increasing popularity, prospective users should always exercise a degree of caution. First and foremost, when a patient has a medical condition that might benefit from any CAM technique, a qualified health care provider should always be consulted before embarking on treatment and even asked about suitable therapists. This is particularly true for pregnant women. Likewise, vigorous massage should be avoided by people with bleeding disorders or low blood platelet counts as well as by patients taking blood-thinners, e.g. aspirin, warfarin and apixaban (Eliquis). Likewise, vigorous massage should be avoided at sites recently operated upon.

Further, although it should be obvious, massage must not be performed on patients with blood clots, open or healing wounds (including sutured skin), skin infections or weak bones (osteoporotic patients). As indicated above, massage therapy and aromatherapy massage may be beneficial with some cancer patients and those undergoing chemotherapies but patients should discuss any proposed CAM technique or treatment with his/her oncologist before receiving treatment. Certainly, application of pressure directly over tumors is unlikely to be recommended or approved.

Before leaving the subject of massage (and aromatherapy) therapy, it might be useful to briefly review the legislative landscape regarding the oils and other products used in these two therapies. Under current U.S. law, the way aromatherapy products are regulated depends primarily on how they are intended to be used based on the labeling and advertising of the products, and the expectations of consumers regarding those products. According to the FDA, if the primary purpose, i.e. the intended use, of a product is to cleanse the body, make the person smell good or to make him or her more attractive, it is classified as a *cosmetic*. Cosmetics as such do not require FDA approval although action can be taken against a marketed cosmetic if there is reliable information showing that it is unsafe when used by consumers in accordance with the directions on the label. Similarly, official action may also be taken if the cosmetic causes problems when used in the customary or expected way as well as if that product is improperly labeled. In contrast to cosmetics, products are classified as *drugs* when intended for therapeutic use, typically preventing or treating disease, or to affect the structure or function of the body, Under the law, drugs must satisfy certain requirements such as FDA approval for safety and effectiveness before they can be marketed.

The FDA ruling is that no medical claims can be made about products that have not been approved by that Agency. This ruling applies to all alternative medicine modalities regardless of effectiveness or their time-honored therapeutic benefits. It is unknown when or even if the FDA or other regulatory bodies will change this situation with many complementary or alternative treatment modalities. Consequently, essential oil suppliers, aromatherapists and other CAM practitioners generally market essential oils as cosmetics and perfumes.

J. A. von FRAUNHOFER

8. ANTIBACTERIAL PROPERTIES OF ESSENTIAL OILS

The word *bacteria* (the singular of which is bacterium) generally has a negative connotation in that bacteria can be dangerous because they are the cause of infections. This blanket disapproval is somewhat misleading because although bacteria can be dangerous (pathogenic), they can also be beneficial, as is the case with the live cultures present in probiotics, yoghurt and other fermented dairy products (see Chapter 4) and those that are involved in such important processes as fermentation for wine making and in various decomposition processes.

Bacteria are usually single cell microscopic living organisms that are found everywhere and especially in living organisms. Vast numbers of bacteria exist within the body and are necessary for the overall health and viability of the human biosystem and over 400 different bacterial species are present in the gastro-intestinal tract (the gut), the skin, the vagina and the oral cavity. In fact, there are over 10^{14} bacterial cells (that is, 1,000,000,000,000,000 cells) in and on the body and their combined weight is about 3.3 lb. (12 kg). In other words, there are about 10 times as many bacterial cells as the total number of cells that make up the human body. The bacteria within the gut perform a variety of functions throughout the entire intestinal system and they are responsible for about 75% of the immune system.

More information on bacteria is provided in Appendix E but, in simple terms, a bacterium is "good" if it contributes to the health of its human (or animal) host or at least is non-pathogenic. On the other hand, a bacterium is "bad" if it is pathogenic or can interfere with the proper function of "good" bacteria.

Until the advent of antibiotics, treating serious skin infections and wounds was not only difficult and often ineffective but, in many cases, the treatment caused as much if not more skin damage than the original wound. This situation changed in the 1940s with the discovery of penicillin and then its later mass production. Thereafter, a plethora of antibiotics and anti-fungal agents became available to successfully treat myriad pathological conditions. Unfortunately, due to overuse and abuse of antibiotics over the past 50 or so years, there has been a proliferation of antibiotic-resistant bacteria, one example of which is MRSA or methicillin-resistant *Staph. aureus*. As a result, treating serious skin infections has become increasingly difficult and there is now a serious lack of antibiotics that can overcome recalcitrant bacterial infections. This has led to a growing interest in alternative and "natural" approaches to treating skin infections and wounds, notably the use of essential oils.[80] This preventive and therapeutic use of essential oils extracted from plants is known as phytomedicine and is a major component of traditional medical practices indicated in Chapter 4.

The essential oils considered in many Online discussions and opinion pieces to have the highest antibacterial activity include eucalyptus, lavender, sage, tea tree oil and thyme. However, documented studies and even quasi-scientific evaluation of the effectiveness of essential oil wound treatments has been lacking for millennia despite the apocryphal effectiveness of essential oils against bacterial infections. This situation changed with the pioneering work of Gattefossé and, later, Valnet in the 20th Century.[81,82,83] These two men probably wrote the earliest monographs on the medical uses of essential oils which, as previously stated, they termed "aromatherapy" (*aromatherapie*).

An incident in 1910 that likely led to Gattefossé's interest in the healing properties of essential oils was the result of a burn to his hands caused by an accident in his laboratory. Apparently, the burn was severe and after the flames were extinguished, gangrene[k] rapidly developed. He applied lavender essence to the burns and within 24 hours, healing started. This antibacterial (and antifungal activity) effectiveness of lavender oil in treating burns as well as insect bites has been confirmed by scientific studies.[84]

Gattefossé continued his investigation of the topical uses of essential oils such as lemongrass oil by treating soldiers in military hospitals during the 1st World War.[1,2,85,86] The French interest in the use of essential oils for medicinal purposes was continued by, amongst others, Jean Valnet. The latter's interest in *aromatherapie* and the healing power of plants apparently stemmed from growing up in a small town on the River Marne in France and seeing that adults knew about, and accepted as a matter of fact, the medicinal properties of many of the local plants. Later, after graduating from medical school, Valnet served in the French army and became Surgeon of the Advanced Surgical Unit at Tonkin, the leading surgical unit in this region of then Indochina (now Vietnam) from 1950–1953. During this time, Valnet found consistent results and had great success in using many essential oils and aromatic solutions to dress wounds. He coined the term *phytotherapy* for his innovative wound treatments. He wrote several books on his treatment approach, some of which are still in use.[87,88,89]

Since the early work of Gattefossé and Valnet, there has been a steady increase in the number of scientific studies of the antibacterial properties of essential oils over several years although, as indicated in Appendix C, the use of oils and perfumes to treat

---

[k] Gas gangrene is a potentially fatal infection of a wound, most commonly by bacterial toxins such as *Clostridium perfringens,* that results in tissue death and subcutaneous swelling and gas. This extremely serious infection was the cause of many amputations and deaths in the First World War on both sides of the conflict.

wounds and infections has been practiced for thousands of years. The EOs that appear to have the oldest and most wide-spread use for health-related purposes are listed in Table 8.1. A quick review of Table 8.1 will confirm how so many of these essential oils are still in everyday use even in the 21st Century. Further, many EOs are used as food preservatives.[90,91]

Table 8.1 Essential Oils Used in Healthcare.

Aniseed	Geranium	Nutmeg
Basil	Juniper	Orange
Camphor	Lavender	Oregano
Cedarwood	Lemon	Peppermint
Cinnamon	Lemongrass	Rosemary
Citronella	Lime	Sage
Clove	Linalool	Tea Tree Oil
Eucalyptus	Mint	Thyme
Frankincense	Myrrh	Wintergreen

Numerous scientific studies have shown that essential oils are rich sources of biologically active compounds and confirmed their bioactivity.[92,14,15,16,17,18] Table 8.2 indicates the bioactivity of many essential oils. Given the bioactivity of many essential oils, it is unsurprising that myrrh was used as a field-dressing for battle wounds by the ancient Greeks and, possibly, the Romans. The work of Gattefossé and Valnet, and more recent evidence,[93] certainly supports the effectiveness of myrrh in wound healing. Perhaps more interesting is that there is now evidence from animal studies that orally-administered myrrh is helpful in gastric ulcer treatment and wound healing.[94]

Table 8.2 Bioactivity of Certain Essential Oils

Antibacterial
Anti-inflammatory
Antimicrobial
Antifungal
Anti-oxidant
Antiseptic
Anti-viral
Insecticidal
Wound healing

These scientific studies indicate that essential oils can be valuable antibacterial agents[95,96] and offer effective treatment for difficult-to-heal wounds[97], plantar warts,[98] nosocomial (hospital-acquired) infections[99] and even multi-drug resistant microorganisms.[100,101] Although some studies indicate that essential oils are effective against fungal infections, this has been questioned by others with regard to treating fungal infections of finger nails and toenails.[102,103] There is also evidence that certain essential oils may be synergistic in their antimicrobial activity, e.g. frankincense and myrrh.[104]

A relative new-comer on the essential oil scene is tea tree oil, also known as melaleuca oil, which is obtained from the leaves of the *Melaleuca alternifolia*, a tree native to Southeast Queensland and the Northeast coast of New South Wales, Australia. Although tea tree oil is toxic when taken by mouth, it shows promise as an antimicrobial agent for many skin infections and dermatologic conditions. These include acne, dandruff, herps, lice and scabies[105,106,107,108,109] as well as being effective in wound healing.[110]

The overwhelming evidence in the scientific literature is that through their bioactivity, essential oils can be used to treat a variety of skin infections and that they can promote wound healing. Nevertheless, this medicinal use of essential oils is not approved by the FDA and, therefore, such healing claims should not be made by suppliers of these products. It should also be noted that because 100% pure essential oils are highly concentrated, they should be used with caution when applied undiluted to the skin. Further, when used for aromatherapy massage, selection of the appropriate essential oil should be made with care to ensure that the patient's skin is not damaged or irritated.[111] This note of caution regarding undiluted essential oil application to the skin comes from the various reports of allergic contact dermatitis experienced by patients and aromatherapists when exposed to essential oils. [112,113,114,] It is possible, however, that these dermatological issues might have been caused or at least exacerbated by adulterants in the essential oil mixtures that were used rather than the essential oil *per se*.

9. KNOWN and LESSER KNOWN ESSENTIAL OILS

Healthcare is rapidly approaching a crisis regarding antibacterials because not only are more and more bacteria developing resistance to antibiotics but the "pipeline" of new antibiotics is virtually non-existent. As a result, many once treatable infections are now recalcitrant and, indeed, can be life-threatening. A good example of this MRSA[1] which responds poorly to a wide variety of antibiotics and is now a serious, potentially life-threatening infection.

Phytomedicine has been used by man almost since the dawn of civilization (see Appendix C) and herbs, spices and essential oils have had a tremendous impact on the health, welfare and the quality of life (QOL) over the millennia.[115] There is increasing interest in the use of natural substances to tackle microbiological assaults on the human body. The greater awareness of the healing potential of essential oils may be because, at least in part, that more and more questions are being raised about the safety of synthetic drugs. This changing attitude by both lay people and medical professionals may result from the fact that the scientific literature provides clear evidence that essential oils extracted from herbs, spices and a wide variety of plants possess strong antimicrobial properties against human and food-borne bacteria and fungi.[116] These herbs/spices

---

[1] Methicillin-resistant *Staphylococcus aureus* (MRSA) infection is caused by a type of staph. bacteria that has become resistant to many of the antibiotics used to treat ordinary *Staphylococcal* infections.

include cinnamon, clove, mint, origanum, salvia and thyme. The antimicrobial and anti-cancer activity of essential oils from botanical sources has been mentioned previously (see Chapters 4 and 8) and is discussed in greater depth below.

There are numerous scientific reports and apocryphal comments regarding the effectiveness of phytomedicine but, nevertheless, many of the therapeutic uses of essential oils are disregarded or unapproved by Government agencies and medical science. The prevailing attitude was that many of the health-related claims for essential oils are "old wives' tales" or urban legends at best. Whereas this may be true in some cases, the body of scientific and clinical evidence suggests otherwise, as indicated by the bibliography cited in this book. The work of Gattefossé and Valnet[80-82,84-89], two of the physicians and scientists who launched *aromatherapie* (see Chapters 5 and 8), should not be dismissed or ignored. There is also a growing body of evidence regarding the antimicrobial and anti-cancer activity of essential oils, as reported here and previously in Chapters 4 and 8.[16-22,91-97,99-101,]

As an interesting example of how ancient folk medicine traditions and modern science support each other, it is worth briefly discussing myrrh, one of the 3 gifts from the Three Wise Men (the Magi) to the baby Jesus. The gift of gold is obvious and so is frankincense because the latter was one of the consecrated incenses described in the Bible and the Talmud. When burned as incense, frankincense emits a fragrant odor and was a symbol of the Divine name as well as an emblem of prayer so that it was an important component of temple services in Jerusalem. It was, consequently, one of the ingredients in the perfume of the sanctuary and was used as an accompaniment to the meal-offering. Since frankincense is often referred to as the "king of oils", that it was a gift to the baby Jesus is unsurprising.

<u>Myrrh</u>

At first sight, the gift of myrrh is curious but when the history of the human use of myrrh is explored and if it is combined with the findings of modern research into the medicinal properties of this essential oil, then this offering is both extraordinary and percipient.

For literally thousands of years, myrrh has been used as incense, an anointing oil and a perfume in many different religions and there are numerous references to these uses in both the Bible and the Talmud. Myrrh, in combination with natron[m], was used for embalming by the Ancient Egyptians as well in the treatment of hay fever and herpes.

Topical use of myrrh is a venerable tradition. The Ancient Greeks and the Romans used it as an antiseptic for treating battle wounds. Traditional Chinese medicine advocated the use of myrrh to treat various joint problems including rheumatism and arthritis as well as for circulatory issues and gynecological problems such as amenorrhea, dysmenorrhea, menopausal pain[n] and uterine tumors. Myrrh has also been an important ingredient in Ayurvedic and Unanic medicine (see Chapter 4) where advantage was taken of the rejuvenating properties of the resin and its curative properties when included in various medicinal formulations. These traditional uses of myrrh are now supported by modern scientific research efforts, both when used alone and in conjunction with frankincense.[94,117]

The antimicrobial properties of myrrh are supported by research studies (Chapter 8). What is perhaps most surprising is that research indicates that myrrh appears to have remarkable preventive and treatment properties with regard to certain cancers, as noted in Chapter 4.

So, modern science supports and validates traditional medicinal uses of myrrh, which is just one of over 300 essential oils. This validation has also prompted modern science to re-examine

---

[m] A naturally occurring mineral that is a mixture of sodium carbonate (Na_2CO_3, soda ash), sodium bicarbonate (baking soda, $NaHCO_3$), salt and sodium sulfate (Na_2SO_4).

[n] Amenorrhea is an abnormal cessation of menstruation whereas dysmenorrhea is the term for painful or difficult menstruation.

other traditional (folk) medicinal practices, as discussed below.

<u>Argan and Jojoba Oils</u>

As mentioned previously in this book, phytomedicine has been used successfully in dermatology for thousands of years. Whereas two essential oils, argan and jojoba, have been used for hundreds of years by Native Americans and tribal communities in North Africa and are familiar components in cosmetics and haircare products for Europeans and Americans, it is only recently that the 100% pure oils have become widely available.

Argan oil is a botanical oil obtained from the kernels of the argan tree (*Argania spinosa* L.) which is endemic to Morocco. Argan oil is produced by traditional methods and is used as both a culinary oil and in cosmetics, notably in haircare products.

Extracting argan oil is a labor-intensive multi-step process. The argan fruit is first dried in the open air and then the fleshy pulp surrounding the nut is removed, usually by hand although some oil producers remove the flesh mechanically without prior-drying of the flesh. In the next stage, the nut is cracked open to free the argan kernels, a process that is performed by hand because it apparently cannot be mechanized. The kernels are then ground and pressed to release pure, unfiltered argan oil which is then decanted into storage vessels. After "resting" for about two weeks during which time solids suspended in the argan oil settle to the bottom of the vessels, the clarified argan oil then is filtered one or more times depending on the requisite final clarity and purity. The approach used to extract argan oil intended for culinary purposes differs slightly in that the argan kernels are gently roasted before they are ground and pressed.

As a culinary oil, notably when used as a dressing for salads and couscous as well as for dipping bread, argan oil has some very interesting and useful properties. It is composed of about 80% unsaturated fatty acids and contains high levels of tocopherols (vitamin E) and carotenes, among many other compounds that promote overall health.[118] As a result, incorporating argan oil in the diet provides many health benefits, including anti-inflammatory effects and, potentially, anti-cancer prevention.[116,119,120,121,122,123] It apparently also has a beneficial impact on rheumatism.

There is also a growing use of argan oil in cosmetics, notably as a skin moisturizer, as a treatment for dry scalp and to impart gloss to the hair as well as naturally repairing the skin barrier.[124] Other topical uses of argan oil include promoting the healing of burns and treating acne vulgaris.°

Jojoba oil is extracted from the seed of the jojoba plant (*Simmondsia chinensis*), a shrub native to Southern California, Southern Arizona and Northwestern Mexico. About 50% of the total seed weight is the oil although the latter is more akin to a mobile wax than a true oil. Because jojoba oil has a very low triglyceride content, it is markedly different from other vegetable oils (see Appendix B).

Jojoba wax (the term commonly being used interchangeably with jojoba oil) has an exceptionally high content of mono-esters of long-chain fatty acids[125] and, consequently has an extended shelf-life and good resistance to decomposition at elevated temperatures. Interestingly, the fatty acid content of jojoba oil varies markedly with several factors, notably the location where the plant is grown (soil and climate) and both the methods used for harvesting and in processing.

Jojoba oil was once used as a substitute for the industrially-important whale oil and has even been used to control powdery mildew plant infections[126] but is now used in its own right as an additive in cosmetics, notably lotions, moisturizers, shampoos and conditioners. It is often used topically on the skin, hair and finger nails and, apparently, Native Americans extracted jojoba oil to treat sores and wounds. A recent review in a leading dermatology

---

° The common names for acne vulgaris include blackheads, skin blemishes, whiteheads and pimples.

journal[127] indicates that jojoba has an anti-inflammatory effect and it can be used on a variety of dermal conditions including skin infections, skin aging, as well as wound healing. Moreover, jojoba has been shown to play a role in cosmetics formulations such as sunscreens and moisturizers and, apparently, it also enhances the absorption of topical drugs.

Essential Oils and Modern Science.

Although essential oils, and complementary and alternative medicine for that matter, are not recognized by the FDA, people use essential oils and alternative medical practices for their health care needs regardless of the law, and will continue to do so for years to come. There are various reasons for this but not the least of which is that people want a more "natural" approach to their health care. Further, because synthetic antimicrobial agents and food additives can cause adverse effects, consumers have a growing interest in both food ingredients and medicinal agents from natural sources, e.g. organic plants, fruits and vegetables. At the same time, there is a growing body of scientific evidence regarding the effectiveness of essential oils in treating a very wide variety of pathological conditions. This is clearly true with regard to the antibacterial action of essential oils and ongoing research supports anecdotal reports of the anti-cancer action of essential oils. Both topics have already been addressed within this book but more recent research has been directed not only at traditional (folk) medicinal practices such as Chinese and Ayurvedic Medicine but also traditional approaches to health care in Lebanon, the Middle East and North Africa. Even more interesting is that essential oils extracted from less common botanical species are also being evaluated for their antibacterial and anti-cancer effectiveness. The rest of this chapter will be devoted to an overview of these research efforts.

<u>Antibacterial activity</u>

It is clear that essential oils and traditional medicine offer considerable promise in treating bacterial infections as well as many other pathological conditions. Many of the essential oils presently being studied for their antimicrobial and anti-cancer (i.e. bioactive) effects are extracted from plants that are less well-known and probably very unfamiliar to Westerners. The antibacterial activity of these "uncommon" essential oils has been the focus of many recent scientific studies, including evaluating their antimicrobial effects against bacteria, yeasts, filamentous fungi, and viruses.[128] The plant sources of these uncommon essential oils are listed in Table 9.1.

Table 9.1 Uncommon Plant Sources of Essential Oils

Species	**Common name**	**Origin**
Aquilaria spp.	Agarwood	China, S.E. Asia, Bangladesh, Tibet
Ballota nigra		Mediterranean region, Central Asia
Bupleurum marginatum		China
Curcuma[1]		China
Guatteria[2]		Amazonia
Lindera		China, East Asia, Eastern North America
Micromeria Bentham		Europe, Asia, Africa, North America
Momordica charantia	Bitter melon, bitter gourd, bitter squash, balsam-pear	India, China
Myrtus communis	Common myrtle	Mediterranean region, North Africa

Nigella[3]	Nigella, devil-in-a-bush, love-in-a-mist	Southern Europe, North Africa, South and Southwest Asia.
Onychopetalum amazonicum R.E. Fr.		Amazonia
Salvia		Middle East
Thymus lanceolatus		Algeria, Tunis
Zornia brasiliensis	Urinária, carrapicho	Amazonia

1: Family of *Zingiberaceae;* 2: Family of *Annonaceae;* 3: Family of *Ranunculaceae*

Two published studies have evaluated the bioactivity of essential oils obtained from curcuma, a common Chinese herb. One study[129] looked at three essential oils (Pian-jiang-huang, Wen-e-zhu, and Wen-yu-jin) extracted from *Curcuma wenyujin*, a traditional medicinal plant in China and the essential oils from the plant are listed in the Chinese Pharmacopoeia. All 3 oils exhibited antimicrobial activity against two bacterial species and one fungal strain but their activities differed, with a greater inhibitory effect being ascribed to one oil (Pian-jiang-huang) which has a higher content of monoterpenes than the others.

A more recent study[130] evaluated the antioxidative, antimicrobial, anti-inflammatory and cytotoxic activities of essential oils extracted from four common but different Curcuma species (*Curcuma longa, Curcuma phaeocaulis, Curcuma wenyujin and Curcuma kwangsiensis*). The oils were tested against the bacteria *E. coli, P. aeruginosa* and *S. aureus*, the yeast *C. albicans* and two cancer cell lines. All 4 essential oils were shown to have antimicrobial, anti-inflammatory (i.e. free radical scavenging capability) and cytotoxic properties. There were differences between the 4 types of essential oils in the bioactivities against bacteria, fungus and cancer cells, the disparities again being ascribed their chemical compositions.

Another herb, *Bupleurum marginatum,* that is indigenous to the southern and southwestern part of China is widely used in many traditional Chinese prescriptions not only has significant *in vitro* antimicrobial activity against Gram positive bacteria[p,q] but also promising anti-inflammatory activity along with strong cytotoxicity against many cancer cell lines.[131]

An essential oil that has been a part of Ayurvedic and Traditional Chinese Medicine for centuries is derived from agarwood[r] and this plant has also been a component of traditional medicine in many countries in South-East Asia, Bangladesh and Tibet. The oil apparently has been used to treat joint pain, inflammatory-related ailments and diarrhea and, evidently, is thought to function well as a stimulant, sedative and cardioprotective agent. Essential oils obtained from agarwood also have complex chemistries and research studies indicate that they exhibit numerous antimicrobial and cytotoxic activities.[132,133] These include antimicrobial, anti-allergic, anti-inflammatory, anti-diabetic, anti-cancer, anti-oxidant and anti-ischemic activities. Interestingly, this essential oil also has a laxative effect and apparently has mosquitocidal properties (i.e. kills mosquitoes).

The Amazon basin is an incredible ecosystem with great biodiversity. It is unsurprising, therefore, that many botanical species indigenous to Amazonia would be the source of essential oils that possess bioactivity. This is certainly true for the *Guatteria* and *Guatteriopsis* species and essential oils distilled from these plants have quite complex chemistries[134] and research studies indicate these essential oils possess antimicrobial activity against 11

---

[p] *Streptococcus pyogenes:* a species of Gram-positive bacteria that is an infrequent, but usually pathogenic, part of the skin flora. Amongst the many ways it can be spread is from cattle to humans through raw milk and contaminated foods.
[q] *Streptococcus agalactiae:* an asymptomatic colonizer of the GI tract in up to 30% of otherwise healthy adults but which, in some circumstances, can cause severe invasive infections.
[r] *Aquilaria spp.*

species of microorganisms.[135] More recent research[136] has not only confirmed this antibacterial effectiveness but also has shown these oils have cytotoxic activity.

The Amazon basin is also the source of other plants whose essential oils possess proven antimicrobial properties. The essential oils obtained from the leaves, twigs and trunk bark of one tree[s] of the genus *Onychopetalum* contains 41 chemical compounds, notably sesquiterpenes and many others. The oils were evaluated for antimicrobial activities against four bacteria strains and five pathogenic fungi and were found to have good activity against *Staphylococcus epidermidis*, *Escherichia coli* and the soil dwelling Gram positive bacterium *Kocuria rhizophila*. [137] Another Amazonian plant, *Zornia brasiliensis* plant, popularly known as urinária, is used in Northeastern Brazilian folk medicine as a diuretic and to treat venereal diseases.[138] Research indicates that the essential oil shows promising cytotoxicity, inhibiting cell proliferation in cultures as well as with the growth of tumors in mice.[138]

Another less common essential oil is obtained from a rare plant species[t] that grows wild in Algeria and Tunisia and which traditionally has been consumed as a beverage and to both flavor and preserve meat and poultry. This particular essential oil contains some 49 different compounds and recent scientific studies showed very promising inhibitory activity against Gram-positive bacteria, especially *Bacillus subtilis*[u] and *Streptococcus pyogenes*[e].[139] This inhibitory activity may be one reason why *Thymus lanceolatus* and its essential oil have been used as a meat preservative. Even more promising is the finding that *in vitro* studies indicate the essential oil is cytotoxic towards 5 different cancer cell lines.[139]

Lebanese folk medicine has traditionally utilized the essential

---

[s] *Onychopetalum amazonicum R.E. Fr. (Annonaceae)*
[t] *Thymus lanceolatus*
[u] *Bacillus subtilis* is found in soil and the gastrointestinal tract of ruminants and humans.

oils from two species of Salvia[v] that are indigenous to the region. The oils have been used to treat microbial infections, cancer, urinary and pulmonary (lung and breathing) problems. Research studies show these oils have good antibacterial activity against Gram-positive bacteria and, surprisingly, an inhibitory effect on human cancer cells by inducing apoptotic cell death.[140] Antimicrobial and anti-oxidative activity[141,142,143] has also been found for three essential oils extracted from other less-common plant species[w] that are indigenous to the Mediterranean region and North Africa.

It follows from the above that once again modern *in vitro* research provides scientific support for the medicinal properties of essential oils from many indigenous plants used in traditional herbal preparations. The other facet of the antibacterial activity of essential oils is that they may offer a solution to the modern threat of increasing bacterial resistance to synthetic antibiotics. Whether bacteria will develop a similar resistance to essential oils has yet to be determined but the fact that they have been used for this purpose for hundreds and if not thousands of years suggests that reduced effectiveness against microbial organisms may not be a problem.

<u>Anti-cancer activity (Cytotoxicity)</u>

The anti-cancer (cytotoxic) activity of essential oils obtained from a variety of botanical sources has been mentioned in Chapter 4 and earlier in this chapter.[134-140] Many other essential oils have also been shown to possess this potentially life-saving property, as discussed below.

Reviews of the scientific literature from nearly 20 years ago and as recently as 2016 clearly show that bioactive phytochemicals in essential oils possess cytotoxic activity, suppressing tumor growth in laboratory (*in* vitro) studies and, interestingly, apparently

---

[v] *Salvia bracteata* and *Salvia rubifolia*
[w] *Micromeria Bentham, Myrtus communis L* and Ballota nigra L. ssp foetida.

may also inhibit cholesterol synthesis in the body.[144,145] Thus, modern research work indicates that traditional (folk) medicinal approaches to treating cancer and many other diseases have a sound and proven scientific basis. What is interesting is that the cytotoxic activity is comparable for essential oil extracted from both wild-grown and cultivated plants. In particular, the essential oils extracted from wild and cultivated *Salvia verbena* showed comparable *in vitro* cytotoxic activity in studies of the inhibition of the growth of cancer cells and the induction of apoptotic cell death.[146]

It has already been stated that essential oils obtained from several plants found in the Amazon basin possess antibacterial activity[134,135] so it is perhaps unsurprising that cytotoxicity properties may be found with other plants from this incredibly diverse ecosystem. Species of one genus of flowering plants from the Brazilian Atlantic Forest[x] are the source of essential oils with complex chemistries. These essential oils not only showed strong antibacterial activity but have been found to exert significant *in vitro* activity against several tumor cell lines and *in vivo* antitumor activity in mice.[147,148] What is particularly significant is that the antiproliferative activity against an ovarian cancer tumor cell line was greater than that the standard chemotherapeutic drug doxorubicin (e.g., Adriamycin® and Rubex®).

Recent studies[149] indicate that essential oils from plant species which are native to southern Europe, North Africa and Southwest Asia, namely nigella, devil-in-a-bush or love-in-a-mist[y], are potential chemotherapeutic and chemo-preventive anti-cancer agents. Another plant that is native to Eastern Asia and the Eastern parts of North America has the common names of spicewood, spicebush, and Benjamin bush[z]. One species, *Lindera strychnifolia*, is widely used in traditional Chinese medicine and studies show that

---

[x] *Guatteria* is in the family *Annonaceae;* note that essential oils from other plants in this family possess antibacterial properties (see references 134 and 135)·
[y] *Nigella* is a genus of 18 species in the family Ranunculaceae.
[z] *Lindera* is part of the *Lauraceae* family

essential oils from this plant also exhibit cytotoxicity and antibacterial activity.[150]

Another plant commonly known as bitter melon or bitter gourd[aa] is cultivated all over the world but notably in tropical areas of Asia, Amazon, East Africa, and the Caribbean. All parts of the plant, including the fruit, are consumed as food and will impart a slightly bitter flavor and taste when cooked with different vegetables in soups or beans. Bitter melon has been used for centuries in Ayurveda medicine (Indian traditional medicine) as a functional food to prevent and treat diabetes and associated complications. Now, recent research[151] has shown that bitter melon has *in vitro* anti-tumor activity when tested against cell lines, inducing cell cycle arrest and apoptosis without affecting normal cell growth. Other research work has confirmed these findings.[152]

Overall, the scientific literature has shown that the many terpenoids and other compounds in essential oils have significant anticancer activities, both on cell lines and on tumors in animals.[153] Not only that, these bioactive constituents of essential oils appear to act synergistically not only with each other but also with conventional chemotherapy and radiotherapy, suggesting that clinical studies in humans should be undertaken.[153]

Just how the anti-cancer (cytotoxic) effects of essential oils operate are unknown but they could involve several different mechanisms. These include antioxidant, antimutagenic and antiproliferative effects, possibly enhancement of immune system functioning as well as enzyme induction and accelerated detoxification, with two or more of these effects working in concert. It should also be noted that since essential oils have complex chemistries and contain a multitude of components, it is probable that there are synergistic effects between many of these constituents. The very complexity of natural essential oils may not only account

---

[aa] *Momordica charantia*

for their bioactivity but also be a warning against expecting synthetic products to exhibit the same efficacy.

<u>Final thoughts</u>

After reading this book, it should be evident that the scientific literature contains a great many research studies confirming the antibacterial and cytotoxic activity of essential oils extracted from numerous herbs and plants. Not only that, modern science clearly validates the effectiveness of a great many CAM and traditional medicinal practices. On the other hand, it has already been mentioned that Governmental agencies and, to a degree, the medical profession are reluctant to recognize the therapeutic value of traditional (folk) medicine. Nevertheless, there is increasing interest in the use of natural substances to tackle microbiological assaults on the human body as well as cancer.

This greater awareness of the efficacy of traditional medical practices and the healing potential of essential oils may be due to several different factors coming into play at roughly the same time. These factors include the growing and alarming resistance of so many different types of bacteria to antibiotics combined with the fact that the safety and often the purity of synthetic pharmaceuticals is increasingly being called into question. Another factor might be that more and more people are looking into the availability of alternative and complementary medical (CAM) practices to treat a variety of medical conditions. This is not just because they have been around for thousands of years but also because the scientific study of both essential oils and CAM therapies has exploded in recent years. There may also be a financial consideration in adopting CAM compared to conventional medical practices. A further consideration is that whereas chemotherapy can be very effective against many types of cancer, there is no escaping the fact that there are many very unpleasant side-effects with these drugs. Whether such side-effects are found with essential oils is unknown but if they do not occur, then there is obviously good reason to explore their use for treating the many and varied forms of this disease.

Finally, it must be stated that although there is so much scientific evidence validating folk medicine and the therapeutic value of essential oils, caution still must be exercised regarding their use, particularly when self-medicating and/or attempting to use them in treating life-threatening diseases. Also, and this is a major reservation, not all so-called 100% pure essential oils are wholly natural products and synthetic "essential oils" may not contain all the minor ingredients present in the natural product. As a result, many of the synergistic effects found with 100% pure natural products may not occur with synthetic oils even though they contain the same principal ingredients.

APPENDIX A. **Atoms and Molecules**

When two or more atoms join or *bond* together, they form a molecule. Compounds are formed when large numbers of molecules bond together and the way these molecules are bonded determines the characteristics of the compound.

When two atoms of hydrogen, oxygen or nitrogen bond to form molecules, they form hydrogen (H_2), oxygen (O_2) and nitrogen (N_2) gases respectively. These are simple molecules. When two atoms of hydrogen and one atom of oxygen bond together, they form water, given the formula H_2O. These individual water molecules can join together in large numbers to form a network in three dimensions which we all recognize as liquid water. When liquid water is heated, the three-dimensional network breaks apart into the individual H_2O molecules and we have the gas known as steam. On the other hand, if liquid water is cooled, the network becomes more stable and rigid, forming ice. When gaseous hydrogen, oxygen and nitrogen are cooled sufficiently, they too form liquids.

Likewise, one carbon atom can bond with two oxygen atoms to form the "greenhouse gas", carbon dioxide with the formula CO_2. When this gas is cooled and pressurized, it forms a liquid which, under further cooling and increased pressure, forms a solid known as "dry ice".

Hydrocarbons and Polymers

Carbon atoms can bond with hydrogen atoms to form what are known as hydrocarbons. The simplest of these is methane or natural gas, with the formula CH_4 indicating that one carbon atom is bonded to 4 hydrogen atoms. Carbon atoms are able to bond together to form chains such as ethane (C_2H_6), propane (C_3H_8) and so on. As the carbon chain or backbone increases in length, i.e. more carbon atoms join together, the resulting molecule gets larger and instead of the hydrocarbons being gases, they become liquids. Thus, the important solvent hexane (C_6H_{14}) has a chain or backbone of 6 carbon atoms and even longer chain hydrocarbons are solids.

Interestingly, chains of carbon atoms and their associated hydrogen atoms can bond or join together to create even longer chains or they form what are known as intermolecular bonds or crosslinks, Figure A.1. The latter effect results in the formation of a fairly stable viscous fluid when enough crosslinks are established between the chains.

Figure A.1 Crosslinking between molecular chains

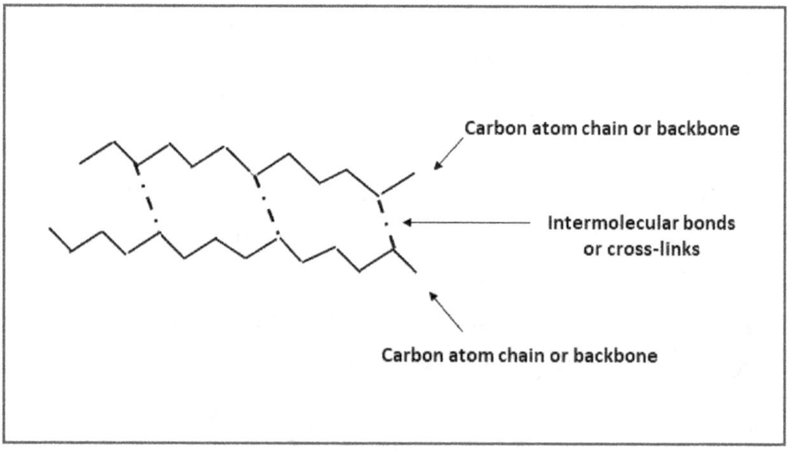

Under pressure or force, e.g. pouring, the crosslinks shift from one atom to another and the chains can slide over each other which, in the case of oils, provides their familiar lubricant action. If the temperature is raised, the crosslinks lengthen and the intermolecular forces decrease so that the oils will become less viscous and flow more easily. When the oil is cooled, however, the crosslinks shorten and bring the chains closer together so that viscosity increases and the oil pours far less readily. If the temperature is decreased enough, the whole mass can become a solid.

When a large number of molecules bond together, typically when long chains of carbon atoms are linked together, a three-dimensional network known as a polymer is formed, where *poly* means many and the word *mer* is short for a molecule. The chains of carbon atoms are referred to as the backbone of the polymer and the process of linking, and crosslinking, of these molecules is known as polymerization. When the chains of polymers are linked or bonded with crosslinks, the network becomes structurally stable and a solid is formed. This is the way plastics such as polyethylene, familiar as plastic bags and wrapping material, are formed.

If atoms such as chlorine or other small molecules replace the hydrogen atoms on the carbon backbone, the polymer becomes more complex and its properties will change. Thus, the polymer known as PVC or polyvinyl chloride, which is formed when chlorine atoms replace every 4th hydrogen atom on the carbon backbone, is more rigid and stronger than the far and simpler polyethylene molecule which only has hydrogen atoms along the carbon backbone. Replacing hydrogen atoms with fluorine atoms produces tetrafluoroethylene or PTFE, commonly known as the anti-stick material Teflon. As the complexity of the parent molecules forming the polymer increases, the properties of that polymer will change, often markedly.

It should be mentioned here, if only for completeness, that other atoms can form networks and polymers. These compounds include silicones which are synthetic (i.e. non-carbon chain) polymeric fluids that have a backbone of alternating silicon and oxygen atoms (...Si$-$O$-$Si$-$O$-$Si...) with organic side chains. The most important of these is polydimethylsiloxane and silicone oils have wide application in industry, typically as lubricants and to produce solid polymers known as silicones. Silicone oils are sometimes added to cooking oils used in deep fat fryers to prevent frothing. In medicine, silicone oils are used in certain ophthalmological situations and may be present in some OTC products for the control of flatulence.

Salts and Esters

Salts are formed when an inorganic acid reacts with a base or alkali. A very common example of this when sodium hydroxide (commonly known as lye) reacts with hydrochloric acid (commonly known as the swimming pool chemical, muriatic acid) to form sodium chloride (table salt):

Sodium hydroxide + Muriatic acid $\longrightarrow$ Sodium chloride
    NaOH   HCl   NaCl

When an organic acid interacts with an alcohol, an ester is formed, an example being the formation of ethyl acetate through reaction between ethanol (ethyl alcohol) and acetic acid (basically vinegar):

    Ethanol + Acetic Acid $\longrightarrow$ Ethyl acetate
    (alcohol)   (acid)   (ester)

As will be seen in the next section, esters known as triglycerides are very important with regard to culinary oils.

Alcohols, Glycerides and Terpenes

If, for example, one hydrogen atom in the simple hydrocarbon molecules methane or ethane is replaced by what is known as a hydroxyl group, i.e., oxygen bonded to a single hydrogen atom (represented as -OH), the resulting compound is known as an alcohol. Thus, when CH_4 is changed or converted to CH_3OH, the latter is known as methyl alcohol or methanol, and when C_2H_6 becomes C_2H_5OH, it is known as ethanol or simply alcohol. The latter is an essential ingredient in beer, wine and liquor.

More complex alcohols are known and an important one is glycerol or glycerin. This has the structure shown on the left in Figure A.2, the OH groups being known as hydroxyls.

Figure A.2 Glycerol and Triglycerides

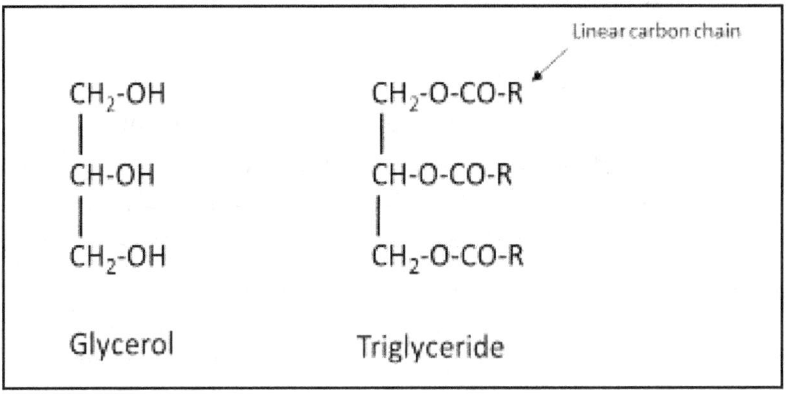

$$CH_2\text{-}OH \qquad\qquad CH_2\text{-}O\text{-}CO\text{-}R \quad \text{Linear carbon chain}$$
$$|\qquad\qquad\qquad |$$
$$CH\text{-}OH \qquad\qquad CH\text{-}O\text{-}CO\text{-}R$$
$$|\qquad\qquad\qquad |$$
$$CH_2\text{-}OH \qquad\qquad CH_2\text{-}O\text{-}CO\text{-}R$$

$$\text{Glycerol} \qquad\qquad \text{Triglyceride}$$

When the -OH (or hydroxyl) group is replaced by larger groups or even long carbon chains, compounds known as triglycerides (meaning all 3 hydroxyl groups in the glycerol have been replaced by carbon chains) are formed. Depending upon the type of molecule or group replacing the -OH group, the properties of the resulting triglyceride can be markedly changed.

Vegetable oils, also known as culinary or cooking oils, are triglycerides in which the carbon chain of the "R" group will be of a different length for each molecule.

In contrast to vegetable oils, essential oils are chemically known as terpenes, a large and diverse class of organic compounds produced by a variety of plants and, particularly, coniferous trees. They are major components of natural resins and, in fact, their name derives from turpentine, the fluid that is distilled from pine resin.

Terpenes are an important class of polymers which are formed when isoprene molecules link together either as chains or as rings, the latter structures being referred to as cyclic, Figure A.3 These structural and compositional differentiations are the source of the well-known differences in color, taste and viscosity between say palm oil and olive oil.

Terpenes are present in almost every living creature and constitute one of the most important "building blocks" in the formation of complex molecules within living organisms and their constituent cells. This process is known as biosynthesis but also as biogenesis or anabolism. There are many examples of the biological importance of terpenes, including Vitamin A and steroids, both of which are derivatives of terpenes.

Figure A.3 Terpenes

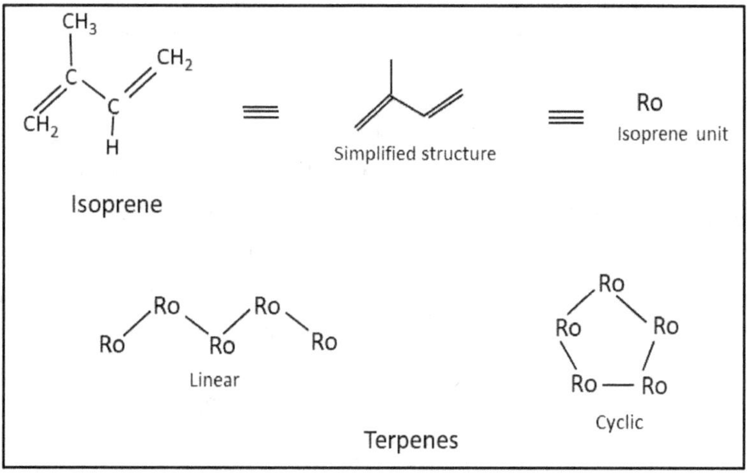

Changes in the size of the terpene backbone or in the atoms attached to the carbon atoms in the basic terpene have a marked effect on the resultant terpenes and compounds derived from them.

When terpenes undergo change after chemical reactions such as oxidation or a rearrangement of the carbon backbone of the terpene molecule, the resultant compounds are known as terpenoids or sometimes as isoprenoids. Many chemists, however, may refer to terpenes and terpenoids collectively as *terpenes*. Because there are chemical differences between terpenes and their associated terpenoids which produced by oxidation and other chemical changes, terpenes and terpenoids will have different properties and characteristics.

Sesquiterpenes, with monoterpenes, are important constituents of essential oils in plants. A particular group of terpenoids, known as sesquiterpenoids are groups of 15 carbon compounds derived or produced by the assembly of 3 isoprenoid units and they are found mainly in higher plants but also in invertebrates. As mentioned in Chapter 4, these compounds are very important with regard to the beneficial health effects of essential oils.

It is clear from this that essential oils, which are often very complex mixtures of terpenes and terpenoids (and many other compounds), will have wholly different compositions, properties, tastes and many other characteristics depending upon their chemical make-up. Further, because heat and reactions such as oxidation can cause changes in the terpene profile and the properties of an essential oil, it follows that careful process control must be exercised when extracting essential oils from their plant sources. The differences in the terpene profiles of essential oils extracted from nominally the same plant that are grown in different locations and even other countries, will effect changes in the final product. This can cause problems and change the characteristics of the resultant product when oils from varied sources are combined into a single batch of "pure" essential oil.

J. A. von FRAUNHOFER

APPENDIX B: **Vegetable Oils**

That vegetable oils have been an important component of human culture almost since the dawn of civilization is clearly evident from numerous Biblical references and many ancient writings. They have been used for millennia as food, cooking media and dietary supplements as well as in a variety of other applications that are unrelated to food. As discussed in Appendix A, vegetable oils are completely different from the other plant-based or botanical oils, essential oils, in terms of their chemistry, characteristics, mode of extraction and their applications.

Vegetable oils, commonly known as cooking or culinary oils, are defined in several different ways but commonly by their source, e.g. nut oils, or their application, notably culinary use, fuel oil and cosmetics. Chemically, most vegetable oils and also animal fats and oils are triglycerides, i.e. tri-esters formed from glycerol and three fatty acid groups (see Appendix A) and these fats are subdivided or classified as being saturated or unsaturated types. Saturated fats, obviously, have no centers of unsaturation, and consequently have relatively high melting points and tend to be solids at room temperature, e.g. cocoa butter. Unsaturated triglycerides, which predominate in vegetable oils, have carbon-carbon double bonds in their backbone. This provides greater reactivity and lower melting points such that these oils are liquids at room temperature.

Vegetable oils, Table B.1, are complex mixtures of a number of triglycerides and this compositional complexity is the source of the different attributes, tastes and uses of these oils. Most oils are extracted from the fruit (seeds) of the plant by pressing, as in the case of olive oil, but sometimes oils may be extracted by pressing the plant leaves. Two other extraction methods also may be used. The first is extraction by immersing the plant material in water or another solvent to leach out the oil and the final product, known as extracted or leached oil, is obtained by evaporating off the solvent. Linseed (flaxseed) oil, for example, is obtained by pressing flaxseed followed by solvent extraction. The second approach to harvesting vegetable oils is liquid-liquid extraction, known as maceration. This involves infusing plant material in a base oil to produce what are known as macerated oils, e.g. extracts of horse chestnuts infused in olive and other oils.

Table B.1 Culinary oils

Almond oil
Avocado oil
Canola (Rapeseed) oil
Cocoa butter (Theobroma oil)
Coconut oil
Corn oil
Cottonseed oil
Flaxseed (Linseed) oil
Grapeseed oil
Olive oil
Palm oil
Peanut oil
Safflower oil
Sesame oil
Soybean oil
Sunflower oil
Walnut oil

A major exception to the extraction methods used for culinary oils is that used for the important (some might say vital) products from the cocoa plant seeds. Once harvested, whole beans are fermented, roasted and then dehusked to leave a residue of cocoa solids. Cocoa butter, also known as theobroma oil, is obtained in what is known as the Broma process which involves hanging bags of roasted cocoa beans at an elevated temperature and collecting the butter that melts out of the beans. In contrast, liquid chocolate extract (chocolate liquor) is produced by pressing out the liquid oil from the solid cocoa residues.

Vegetable oils and health

The health claims of vegetable oils are based on their naturally low content of saturated and trans fats and the high (and healthier) unsaturated fat contents, especially the omega-3 fatty acid ALA (α-linolenic acid).

The Internet is replete with countless claims for the health benefits of vegetable oils; some of these claims are supported by the scientific literature but many are simply apocryphal and, in some cases, may be wishful thinking. In fact, FDA regulations currently ban heart-health claims in labeling for many cooking oils and vegetable oil spreads, in part to discourage such claims in advertising. One reason for this is that heart-health claims can promote the misperception that these products are healthy in all respects. In fact, many culinary oils may have high total fat and calorie contents which, in turn, can result in weight gain and associated heart problems.

Basically, when packaging nutrient content claims such as "low in saturated fat" or "no trans fats" are made, they generally have little impact on consumer awareness of the caloric content of the products. This can lead to the perception that the vegetable oil-based products are beneficial to health in every respect. Clearly, there is a very real need for greater consumer awareness regarding the caloric content of cooking oils since even small changes in caloric intake, regardless of the source, can have long-term effects on weight gain and the heart (cardiac) health of consumers.

APPENDIX C. **Historical perspective**

Essential oils and perfumes (as well as spices) have been around since the dawn of civilization but ancient oils and extracts most certainly did not have anything like the purity or potency of what is available now. Not only that, extracting essential oils from their parent plants was considerably less efficient than is possible today. It is not clear how essential oils were obtained in early times but it is possible that the method known as *enfleurage* or maceration was used back in Biblical times. Enfleurage is still practiced today in Europe and elsewhere (see Chapter 3) although distillation is used considerably more widely for obtaining essential oils and with greater efficiency.

Historical records suggest that the art of distillation was described by Herodotus about 400BC and then again, some 50 years later by Aristotle. However, the discovery of earthenware distillation apparatus dating back to about 3000 BC suggests that steam distillation to extract essential oils may have been practiced for some 5000 years. Archeological findings and written records indicate that crude distillation techniques were developed by Greek chemists in Alexandria in the 1st Century AD and in China during the Han Dynasty (100-200 AD). However, it should be noted that it is possible that the primary purpose of such distillation techniques was to produce alcoholic beverages, purified water and so-called divine water, digestive tonics and medicinal fluids rather than just essential oils.

Since those very early days, there have been written records of distillation of water and essential oils that have continued until the present day. These early references include Arabian chemists in the 1st and 2nd Centuries AD and Zosimus of Panopolis in the 5th Century AD. There have also been sporadic comments about practicing rudimentary distillation during the Dark Ages (the early Middle Ages) and, apparently, slightly more refined techniques were developed in China during the Jin (12th–13th centuries), Southern Song (10th–13th centuries) and Yuan (13th-14th centuries) dynasties. Since then, of course, distillation methods have become far more efficient, better controlled and based upon science rather than trial-and-error methodologies. In addition to the greater efficiency and through-put performance of modern distilleries, superior construction materials and manufacturing technology both have greatly reduced the inclusion of impurities in essential oils due to the processing equipment.

The antiquity of essential oils, aromatics and the healing properties of oils, herbs and plants is well established by numerous ancient documents and records. It should be mentioned, however, that although perfumes, salves, lotions and many other medicinal concoctions have been known for literally thousands of years, the medicinal potency of these medications was probably somewhat limited. The word *perfume*, for example, had a far broader meaning in Ancient Times than today and covered not just perfume but also incense, spices, ointments and drugs. The origin of the word perfume is thought to be the Latin phrase *per furnum* (by or through fire or an oven). This may be a reference to obtaining essential oils by distillation or the spiritual role of perfumes in the sacrificial fires intended to provide food for the gods who would starve without these offerings.

Historically, most perfumes were obtained from herbs, bushes or trees although a few were derived from animal sources. Many of these aromatics were obtained or harvested by wounding or "tapping" trees and the base or principal ingredient for the perfume either trickled out or simply oozed out of the wound. This method, albeit refined, is still used for harvesting the sap from maple trees for making maple syrup. A further source of these oleoresins was the accumulation or accretion of substances beneath a bruise in the bark. These substances were not the sap of the tree and despite their chemical complexity, these oleoresinous components fell into three main groups:

1. Resins: insoluble in water but often soluble in alcohol,
2. Gums: insoluble in alcohol but capable of absorbing water to form a mucilage (an aqueous viscous fluid), and
3. Oleoresins and balsams: solutions of resins in volatile oils and the primary source of perfumes.

The quantity of different resins, gums and balsams used in antiquity was enormous in both the number of varieties and amount of material but the most important were frankincense, myrrh and turpentine, all of which were obtained from trees of those names. Of these, myrrh was the most widely used although the proportion used for medical purposes is unknown There was also another substance known as mastich, derived from the lentisk shrub. Mastich softened readily in the mouth and was probably both the chewing gum of the old world and the origin of the medical term *masticate* (to chew).

Traditionally, frankincense was collected by making longitudinal incisions through the bark and allowing the white gum to come to the surface where it solidified. Within 1-2 weeks, the white lump dried into an amber-colored oleoresin gum that ignites easily and gives off a pleasant smell (i.e., incense). In contrast, the bark of the myrrh tree apparently cracks spontaneously, allowing the oleoresin to trickle out and eventually harden into a reddish-brown mass. Myrrh has a characteristic bitter taste and its name derives from the Hebrew and Arabic word *murr* for bitter.

This ancient use of balsams (the aromatic resinous substances exuded by various trees and shrubs) as a base for certain fragrances and medical and cosmetic preparations as well as to treat wounds has a number of overtones. There might have been a conscious or perhaps an unconscious analogy between the healing powers of gums exuded by trees to heal injuries or wounds in their bark and the use of these gums for human wounds. Secondly, infected wounds smelt bad and the perfume or aroma of oleoresins not only eliminated the odor but helped the curative process and, for example, Theophrastos in 300 B.C. provided the formula of a perfume containing burnt resin, cassia, cinnamon and myrrh that was intended to relieve wound inflammation. Thirdly, resins are one of the few products in nature that never decay and the ancients might have considered that this characteristic was transmissible to wounds.

There are numerous references to oils and perfumes throughout both the Old and New Testaments of the Bible. Within roughly the same time period, the large body of knowledge originating in the ancient Indian subcontinent, writings known as the Vedas and dating from about 2000 BC, compiled lists of medicinal plants and aromatics. Ancient Egypt, notably Eber's Papyrus, which dates from about 1550 BC and believed to have been copied from other written work as old as 3400 BC, likewise itemized medicinal plants and aromatics. This knowledge apparently was acquired by Democrates and Heodotus, who visited Egypt around 425 BC, and this information then spread throughout Ancient Greece. It is not clear when aromatic oils became established throughout Arabia but Arabian frankincense and myrrh, both of which have far superior aromas were of considerably greater antiquity than what the Greeks and Egyptians customarily used. The Ancient Egyptians imported huge amounts of Myrrh as early as 2500 B.C., although the proportion used for medical purposes is unknown. There are also numerous references in ancient papyri to resin-based wound salves and in 1370 B.C. Milkili, one of the lieutenants of the Egyptian pharaoh Amenophis IV (also known as Akhenaten), wrote to the pharaoh asking for myrrh to use in treating battle casualties.

The Ancient Greeks used aromatic plants and bushes, principally the turpentine tree, for incense and to treat wounds. Herodotus, for example, referred to the use of myrrh to tend the captain of a Greek trireme who suffered severe wounds in a naval battle around 480 BC. Hippocrates (460-370 BC), the "father" of organized medicine, used aromatic vapor for inhalation to treat disease and frequently prescribed myrrh to treat various conditions, including bacterial infections.

The Ancient Romans also were familiar with aromatic oils and archeology indicates that they used scented oils for a variety of purposes including massage. Apparently, the Roman physician Celsus used a wine-myrrh lotion to treat bums around 100 AD. The Inner Cannon of China's Yellow Emperor, compiled 475-200 BC, also listed a wide variety of medicinal plants and aromatic oils although their precise identities are unknown.

Perfumes and aromatic oils were considered to be basic necessities of life in Biblical times. It is stated in the Old Testament of the Bible that *ointment and perfume rejoice the heart* while there are comments by historians that slave laborers (and probably the Israelites) in Ancient Egypt sometimes went on strike because their food was bad and they no *ointment* to improve the taste. Based on the history of oleoresins and essential oils, it would appear that two of the gifts of the Three Wise Men to the infant Jesus Christ had greater significance than merely their scarcity and cost. The offering of gifts that had both spiritual and medical overtones, particularly their usefulness in wound treatment and healing of various pathological conditions, makes sense in the light of the medical and hygienic aspects of the Jewish Talmud and the Old Testament. Expertise in wound healing was likely essential given the necessary warlike nature of the ancient tribes of Israel.

After the fall of the Roman Empire and the start of the so-called The Dark Ages, namely the early Middle Ages from about 460 to 1000 AD, the use of aromatics was strictly curtailed and the Catholic Church even deemed bathing to be decadent if not sinful. At the same time, the Church also dismissed the holistic health-care and medical principles of Hippocrates and healers who used essential oils, perfumes and herbs for their curative properties were often condemned for witchcraft and burned at the stake. It appears, however, that the art of essential oil extraction (i.e. distillation) and their use in medicine and aromatherapy was continued in some secrecy by monks within their cloistered communities. This covert action apparently also applied to herbal medicine although it is possible, and highly likely, that aromatic oils and spices were used as air fresheners to offset the malodorous emanations from unwashed bodies.

This situation continued until the advent of the Renaissance or the Age of Enlightenment (14th – 17th centuries). This period in history was when personal hygiene and the use of essential oil and other plant-based remedies for medicine (and enhancing the quality of life) was once again deemed acceptable, if not necessary. Many physicians became adept at treating a wide variety of diseases and bacterial skin infections using herbal and plant-based (essential oil-containing) medicines, and probably prevented the spread of a great number of devastating diseases. The ability of plant extracts to improve the course of wound healing became both widespread and acceptable, and even Guido Majno, in his book on wound healing in the Middle Ages, refers to a simple bacteriological study in which myrrh was tested against a selection of bacteria. It was found that myrrh dissolved readily in water and that it acts as a bacteriostatic agent against *Staphylococcus aureus* (a common wound bacterium and the cause of osteomyelitis, a frequently intractable bone infection) and other Gram positive bacteria. In other words, myrrh appears to have a comparable antibacterial effect to the modern antibiotic, penicillin and later antimicrobial drugs. A sister compound of frankincense and myrrh is still used by African herbalists to treat genito-urinary problems, particularly persistent barrenness and male impotence.

By the 1600's, writings about herbal medicine and essential oils became widespread. By the 1800's most of the pharmacopoeia of England, Germany and France were referencing and prescribing essential oils for a variety of illnesses. At the same time, large flower-growing districts in the south of France were supplying raw materials for French perfumers. Tuberculosis was common, yet workers processing flowers and herbs generally remained disease-free and this prompted some of the early laboratory-based or *in vitro* studies of the antibacterial properties of essential oils. More recent studies over the past few years have confirmed that various essential oils, including citrus oil, citronellol, linalool and eucalyptol oil, can inhibit airborne tuberculosis transmission by more than 90 percent.

It was in the early 1900s that essential oils (and their derivatives, perfumes) became established and recognized for their effectiveness in wound healing and for other health benefits rather than simply for their pleasing aromas. In 1910 Rene-Maurice Gattefossé, a French cosmetic chemist, severely burned his hands and arms in an accidental lab explosion. He extinguished the flames but as he described it, "both my hands were covered with rapidly developing gas gangrene." He treated his burns with lavender oil, reporting that "just one rinse with lavender essence stopped the gasification of the tissue. This treatment was followed by profuse sweating and healing which began the next day."

Although he previously had no interest in natural healing methods, his astonishing burn experience led Gattefossé to investigate the medical uses of essential oils by treating soldiers in military hospitals during World War I. He coined the term "aromatherapie" in 1920's-1930's – the treatment of disease and injury using aromatic essential oils. Another Frenchman, Jean Valnet, a Parisian physician and army surgeon, began to use essential oils with great success as antiseptics and anti-microbials when treating war wounds during the Indochina war from 1948-1959. As the story goes, he was stationed in Indochina (now Vietnam) and treating war wounded soldiers when he ran out of his supply of antibiotics. Out of desperation he began to use essential oils on the injured. He was amazed to see how the essential oils fought infection, crediting many lives saved due to the use of essential oils. After the war, he continued using essential oils in his private medical practice and published in 1964 the comprehensive textbook *The Practice of Aromatherapy*. This monograph earned Valnet global recognition and stimulated further interest in, and the continuing investigation of, the curative properties of essential oils.

In the 1980's the French physician, Daniel Pénoël, and his colleague, the biochemist Pierre Franchomme, investigated and catalogued the medical properties of over 270 essential oils. In 1990, they co-authored a reference book, *L'aromatherapie Exactement*, that listed the medicinal properties of essential oils and the book soon became the primary reference work for later researchers investigating the medical benefits of essential oils.

It is clear that there is a lesson to be learned from this historical perspective of essential oils for the modern physician and healthcare provider, particularly for those concerned with immediate (triage) treatment of wounds and similar injuries. The properties of myrrh, and presumably those of many other oleoresins, appear to make them very useful components of emergency medical kits and as well as adjunct antibacterial agents. In other words, because resins do not decay and they can be activated by dissolution in water, myrrh and similar ancient *perfumes* may be effective antibacterials without the limited shelf-life of modern antibiotics and, possibly, their effectiveness may not be limited by the increasing common, and very worrying, bacterial resistance found with modern antibiotic therapy.

APPENDIX D. **Distillation**

Before discussing distillation, the predominant means of extracting essential oils from botanicals, it might be interesting to look at the history of distillation because, like essential oils themselves, it is a process steeped in history.

<u>History of Distillation</u>

Historical records suggest that the process of distillation was first described by Herodotus about 400 BC and then again, some 50 years later, by Aristotle. However, the discovery of earthenware distillation apparatus dating back to about 3000 BC suggests that the tradition of extracting essential oils by distillation and perhaps distillation of liquors may have been practiced for some 5000 years.

Archeological findings and written records indicate that Greek chemists in Alexandria in the 1st Century AD developed crude distillation techniques as did "chemists" in China during the Han Dynasty (100-200 AD). However, it should be noted that it is possible that the primary purpose of such distillation techniques was to produce purified water and so-called divine water, alcoholic beverages, digestive tonics and medicinal fluids rather than just essential oils. Other early references to distillation include Arabian chemists in the 1st and 2nd Centuries AD and the Greek-Egyptian chemist, Zosimus of Panopolis in the 5th Century AD. Slightly more refined distillation techniques, primarily for beverages, were developed in China during the Jin (12th–13th centuries), Southern Song (10th–13th centuries) and Yuan (13th-14th centuries) dynasties.

Records indicate sporadic comments were made about

rudimentary distillation being performed in Europe and elsewhere during the Dark Ages (the early Middle Ages). Apparently. distillation of alcohol was performed in the 12th Century at the School of Salerno, the original location of the European Medical School, and fractional distillation apparently was developed by Tadeo Alderotti, an Italian doctor and professor of medicine at the University of Bologna, in the 13th Century. The German alchemist, Hieronymus Braunschweig, wrote the first treatise on distillation, *Liber de arte destiilandi* (Book of the Art of Distillation), in 1500 which he revised and expanded in 1512. Apparently, this book is thought to be the basis for the first major compendium on distillation in the English written language by John French in 1651.

Most of these early approaches to distillation would appear to be based on alchemy and used much the same apparatus. Alchemy was, and still is to some degree, a philosophical and protoscientific tradition practiced throughout Europe, Egypt and the Middle East, and Asia. It aims to purify, mature and perfect certain objects. Within the history and philosophy of science, protoscience has several meanings but basically it refers to early scientific studies starting in the 17th Century which were practiced by interested individuals who were largely self-educated and did not have access to scientific information and had to establish for themselves the verifiable principles and laws that still exist today. Even that scientific giant of the late 17th and early 18th Centuries, Sir Isaac Newton, whose laws of physics and calculus are still in use today, was an alchemist and a protoscientist. Interestingly, Newton, in addition to watching apples fall and quantifying gravity as well as the laws of motion, also spent time and energy attempting to transmute base metals such as lead into gold, a practice known as chrysopoeia.

The earliest distilling apparatus was the alembic, see the figure below (https://upload.wikimedia.org/wikipedia/commons/7/79/Alembic.jpg).

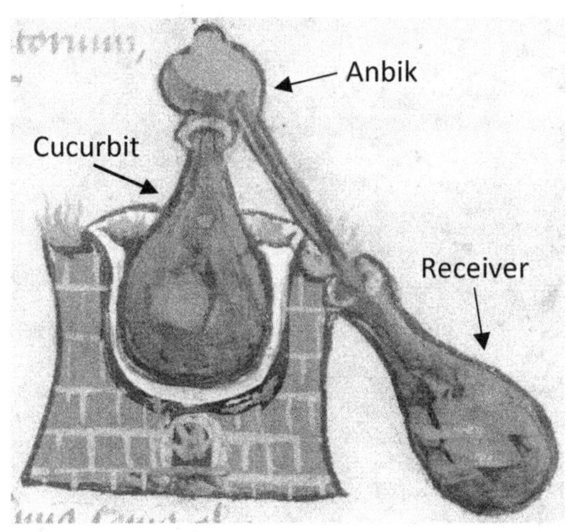

It comprised three parts, the cucurbit, the anbik (the head or cap), and a receiver.

The cucurbit or still pot holds the liquid to be distilled and is heated. The head or cap (the anbik) fits over the cucurbit and the vapor from the cucurbit liberated by heat rises into it. Attached to the head is a tube that slopes downward so that the condensed vapor or distillate feeds fed into the receiver. Also, with advances in the available materials for fabricating the equipment, vapor condensation became more efficient by cooling both the delivery tube and the receiver.

Over time, the alembic morphed into a device known as a retort which had the cucurbit and anbik built into a single unit. Originally, retorts were made from metal such as copper but with the greater availability of glass and improved glass-blowing techniques, most retorts were made of glass. Also, glass retorts were less reactive than metal, so that the distillate was purer and free of contaminants leached from the metal or the earthenware of the alembic. Further, it was possible to use running water to cool the receiver, something that was not always possible with the earthenware alembics due to the risk of cracking.

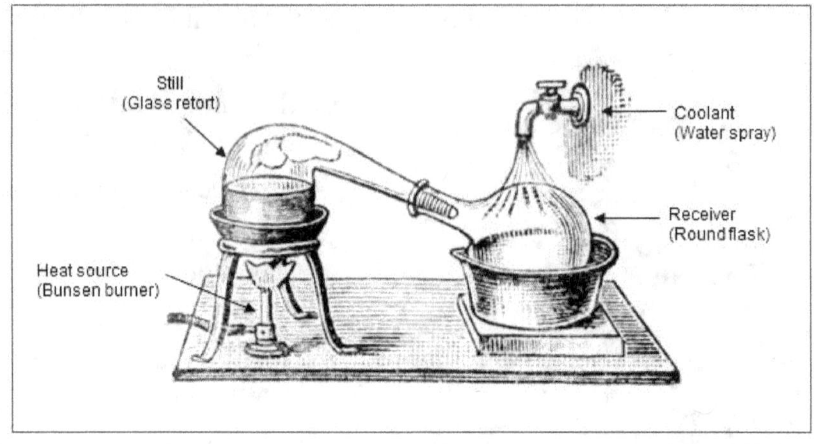

Schematic diagram of a glass retort in use.
(https://upload.wikimedia.org/wikipedia/commons/1/17/Distillation_by_Retort.png)

A modern descendant of the alembic (and the glass retort) is the pot still, a device used to produce distilled beverages (liquors such as whisky, brandy, vodka, etc. as well as "moonshine") and, to some degree, essential oils.

The basics of modern distillation techniques were established by the early to mid-19th century and innovations/improvements such as pre-heating, reflux condensation and continuous stills were developed and improved upon by many scientists and engineers. When chemical engineering became established as a recognized discipline at the end of the 19th century, more science was injected into distillation and empirical methods were largely dismissed. Further advances in distillation came about by the development of the modern petrochemical industry, which started in 1920 and led to improved fractionation methods and, later, the use of computer simulation of the fractional distillation process to improve yields and product purity from crude oils.

Since those early days, of course, few people practiced alchemy and distillation methods have become far more efficient, better controlled and based upon science rather than trial-and-error methodologies. In addition to the greater efficiency and through-put performance of modern distilleries, the availability of superior construction materials and advances in technology have greatly reduced the inclusion of impurities in essential oils due to the processing equipment.

Basics of Distillation

Distillation is simply a process by which one or more components of a liquid mixture are separated by selective evaporation and condensation. It involves heating the liquid mixture to force at least one of the components into the gas phase and the gas is then collected at the top of the still and cooled to condense it back into liquid form which is then collected in a suitable receiver. When the process is repeated on the collected liquid to increase the purity of the product, it is called double distillation. By its very nature, distillation is a physical separation process not a chemical reaction, and this distinguishes it from other methods used to extract essential oils from plants, e.g., enfleurage.

Depending upon the conditions and the method used, distillation can completely separate the individual components in a mixture to yield pure compounds or may only accomplish a partial separation that increases the concentration of selected components within the starting mixture. In either case, the process involves the differences in the volatility of the components in the original mixture. Volatility is the rate at which a chemical compound will evaporate; it increases with temperature and decreases with the atmospheric pressure or the pressure within the distillation unit. Atmospheric pressure can markedly influence volatility and, for example, water boils at temperatures far below 212°F (100°C) at high altitudes due to the lower atmospheric pressure. In other words, distillation is a process used to separate mixtures based on the temperature differences required to change the phase, i.e., from liquid to gas, of the components within the mixture. This means that for multi-component mixtures, the various substances in the mixture are evaporated at different pressures and different temperatures and that is the basis for their separation.

Various types of distillation can separate the components in a mixture, including simple, continuous, fractional, vacuum, flash, solar, vapor and destructive distillation. Distillation is used for many commercial processes, such as the production of gasoline, kerosene and many organic solvents and petrochemicals from crude oil. Further, gas mixtures may be liquefied and separated; nitrogen, oxygen, and argon for example are distilled from air. Most of these distillation methods are important in both the chemical laboratory and in industry but are not really pertinent to the essential oil industry and need not be discussed further here

The primary focus in both laboratory scale and industrial distillation is purification. In contrast, distillation performed for beverages (e.g. liquors) and in essential oil extraction does not have the objective of true purification but the transfer of all volatiles from the original mixture to the distillate. That is why distillers of essential oils often refer to their work as more of an art than a science because it requires considerable skill to capture all the "essentials" in an essential oil without damaging the product or losing components.

Simple Distillation

In simple distillation, a mixture is heated to change the most volatile component from a liquid into vapor within a containing vessel or still. This, as mentioned above, is known as volatilization. The less volatile component, with a higher boiling point than that of the compound being volatilized off, remains behind in the mixture. The vapor released by volatilization rises and is passed into a condenser. Usually, the condenser is cooled, typically by a surrounding jacket that has running cold water passing through it; this cooling promotes condensation of the vapor, which is collected. Simple distillation can be used to separate liquid mixtures, liquids from solids or volatile liquids from nonvolatile components also present in the original mixture.

Simple distillation is used when the components to be separated in the liquid (mixture) have several common properties. In particular, the liquids should be relatively pure, contain less than 10% contaminants and, ideally, the contaminating liquid should have a boiling point that is 50-70°C (122-158°F) greater than that of the desired distillation product. If the difference in boiling points of the components in the liquid is not large, i.e., less than 50-70°C, simple distillation may not be an effective method of separating them. In such cases, the more complex and industrially important process of fractional distillation has to be used to achieve component separation.

Initially, most distillations were batch processes using one vaporization and one condensation with purity being improved by further distillation of the condensate. Greater volumes were processed by simply repeating each distillation with new material or redistilling condensates. Apparently, ancient distillers and artisans performed as many as 500-600 distillations in order to obtain a pure compound.

Steam Distillation

Steam distillation used to separate heat-sensitive components and involves passing steam into the mixture, causing heating of the mixture and some of it to vaporize. This vapor is cooled and condensed into two liquid fractions. Sometimes the fractions are collected separately or, because they have different densities, they separate on their own. In common with vacuum distillation (see below), steam distillation is a method of achieving distillation at temperatures lower than the normal boiling point of the component to be separated.

Steam distillation often is used when the component to be distilled is immiscible (incapable of mixing) with, and chemically unreactive, with water. This separation effect occurs when flowers (botanicals) are steam distilled and the distillation products are the essential oil and a water-based (aqueous) distillate.

Vacuum Distillation

Vacuum distillation is used to separate components in a mixture when the components have high boiling points. Lowering the pressure within the still also lowers boiling points, as noted above. In most other respects, vacuum or reduced pressure distillation is essentially the same as other (simple) distillation methods.

This distillation method is particularly useful when the normal boiling point of a compound is greater than its decomposition temperature, i.e., the compound to be separated will be damaged or decomposed by the temperature of steam, boiling water or the heat required to volatilize it. These are important considerations in petrochemical processing. Whereas this methodology does have a somewhat higher operating cost, there is a lower capital cost for the construction of the distillation column. Further, because the temperatures involved in vacuum distillation are lower, there is a reduced risk of product degradation, an important factor in the petrochemical industry, the overall process improves separation because of greater capacity, higher yields and superior product purity.

Fractional Distillation

When the components of a mixture have boiling points and volatilities that are close to each other, they are separated by what is known as fractionation or fractional distillation. The underlying basis for this approach is the same as for simple distillation except that the process is repeated many times within a single unit. Although fractionation is rarely used for essential oils, it is mentioned here of it for the sake of completeness.

When simple distillation is performed on a mixture of liquids with similar volatilities, the resultant distillate will have a higher level of the more volatile compound than the original mixture but it would still contain a significant amount of the higher boiling compound. If the distillate from the first simple distillation is redistilled, as in double distillation, there will be a higher content of the lower boiling compound but the distillate would still contain some of the higher boiling compound. Although repeating this process many times would eventually yield a fairly pure distillate, it would take a long time and be wasteful of resources and this is where fractional distillation comes in.

The primary difference between the equipment used in simple distillation and that in fractional distillation is that in the latter, a packed fractionating column is attached to the top of the distillation vessel between it and the condenser/collector. As the mixture in the still is heated, vapor rises and enters the fractionating column. The packing within the column has a large surface area and as the rising vapor from the still cools, it condenses on the packing material. The heat of more rising vapor causes this liquid to vaporize again, moving it along the column. As vapors continue to rise through the column, the liquid that has condensed will revaporize. Each time this occurs, the content of the more volatile substances increases in the resulting vapors. The length (or height as these columns are usually built vertically) of the fractionating column and the packing material determine the number of times the vapors will re-condense before passing into the condenser; the number of condensations is referred to as the number of theoretical plates of the column.

In other words, the fractionating column separates the components in a series of distillations called rectification. The fractionating column is heated so that there is a temperature gradient down the column. Ideally, the temperature in the distillation flask would be equal to the boiling point of the mixture of liquids and the temperature at the top of the fractionating column is that of the boiling point of the lowest boiling compound. If this can be achieved, all of the lowest boiling compound would be distilled away before any of the higher boiling compound reaches the top of the column. In reality, fractions of the distillate must be collected because as the distillation proceeds, the concentration of the higher boiling compound in the collected distillate steadily increases. Fractions of the distillate, which are collected over a small temperature range, will be essentially purified; several fractions are collected as the temperature changes and these portions of the distillate are re-distilled to increase the purification that has already occurred.

APPENDIX E: **Bacteria**

Bacteria are microscopic living organisms, usually one-celled, that are found everywhere. They can be dangerous, such as when they cause infection (pathogenic bacteria), or beneficial, such as those present in probiotics, yoghurt and the bacteria involved fermentation processes (such as in wine making) and that of decomposition.

Bacteria have different shapes and may be spherical, spiral or rod-shaped and are present singly or in chains; they are named after their shapes. Rod bacteria, as the name implies, are microbial species with the shape of a rod. A coccus (plural: cocci) is a type of bacterium that has a spherical or ovoid shape. A cluster of bacteria with the appearance of a bunch of grapes is designated "staphylococci" whereas chains of clustered bacteria are called "streptococci". Many cocci but certainly not all are pathogenic, causing a variety of diseases such as "strep. throat", pneumonia, meningitis, gonorrhea and rheumatic fever, to name but a few.

In microbiology, the term "colony forming unit" or CFU is often used. This term refers to a common laboratory procedure in which a small amount of microbial matter is spread over the surface of a suitable culture or growth medium gel in a plate known as petri dish, which is then placed in an incubator. After a set period of time, the number of colonies (growing clumps of bacteria) will equal the number of viable organisms in the sample. The appearance of the CFUs and certain other characteristics are used to identify the species under examination.

Finally, a word about bacterial nomenclature. The name of the genus or family of bacteria is italicized and followed by *spp.*, e.g. *Bifidobacterium spp.* refers to the genus of Bifidobacteria that resides in the healthy human digestive tract. Commonly, in microbiology, the name of a particular genus of bacteria is shortened to a single capital letter, usually italicized, with a second word indicating which species is under discussion. For example, *Escherichia coli* is commonly referred to as *E. coli*, *Escherichia* being the genus and *coli* the species.

Gram-positive and Gram-negative bacteria

Bacterial species may be classified as being Gram-positive or Gram-negative. This classification system and method of identifying bacteria by staining was developed by the Danish physician and bacteriologist, Hans C. J. Gram, and is based on the chemical and physical properties of their cell walls. Because of differences in the cell walls of the bacteria, a Gram-positive (also written as Gram+) bacterium acquires a purple/blue color in Gram's staining method whereas a Gram-negative (also written as Gram-) bacterium takes on a pink/red color. Although most bacteria are either Gram-positive or Gram-negative, there are a few other types, known as Gram-variable bacteria, that yield a mixture of colors in Gram's staining method and yet others, known as Gram-indeterminate bacteria, which do not respond to Gram staining at all.

Gram-negative bacteria

The vast majority (some 90-95%) of Gram-negative bacteria are pathogens and are harmful to the body whereas most Gram-positive bacteria are non-pathogenic and may be beneficial to health.

The major cause of the pathogenicity of Gram-negative bacteria is the structure of the cell membrane. When the cell wall breaks down, a bacterial toxin known as an endotoxin within the body of a bacterium is released. If the endotoxin enters the bloodstream and can then reach any part of the body, it can cause a pathological effect such as a toxic reaction. The symptoms of a toxic reaction may be that the sufferer will develop a high temperature (known as a pyrogenic effect), an accelerated respiration rate and low blood pressure, and this sometimes may lead to fatal endotoxic shock.

Although millions of Gram-negative bacteria are present in the gut, endotoxin released by these bacteria is detoxified and eliminated by the liver in healthy individuals. However, if the level of endotoxin increases beyond that which can be detoxified by the liver and starts spreading through the body, the immune system releases an inflammatory substance and causes the body temperature to rise and fight the infection. When the levels of endotoxin in the blood rise above that which can be controlled by the immune system, endotoxic shock can occur. When an antibiotic that can work against Gram-negative bacteria is administered, it is essential that the patient complete the prescribed course of antibiotics both for the antibiotics to work properly and to stop the Gram-negative bacteria from developing resistance to these antibiotics.

Table D.1 *Principal Gram-negative bacteria and associated diseases*

Genus	Species	Disease caused
Bordetella	*B. pertussis*	Whooping cough
Brucella	*Br. abortus*	Undulant fever
Escherichia	*E. coli*	Cystitis, pyelitis, suppuration
Hemophilus	*H. influenza*	Meningitis, conjunctivitis, influenza
Klebsiella	*K. pneumonia*	Pneumonia*
Neisseria	*N. meningitides*	Cerebrospinal meningitis
Proteus	*P. vulgaris*	Suppuration
Pseudomonas	*P. mallei*	Glanders
	P. aeruginosa	Suppuration
Salmonella	*S. typhosa*	Typhoid fever
Shigella	*S. dysenteriae*	Bacillary dysentry
	S. paratyphi	Paratyphoid fever, gastroenteritis

Vibrio	*V. comma*	Cholera
Yersinia	*Y. pestis*	Plague

Gram-Positive Bacteria

The most important forms of Gram-positive bacteria are bacilli (rod-shaped microorganisms) and cocci (spherical or ovoid in shape). Certain Gram-positive bacteria are pathogenic but there are many more that are beneficial to the human body, i.e. they are "good" bacteria, as often mentioned in regard to probiotics.

Bifidobacteria spp. are Gram-positive anaerobic (see below) bacteria that are one of the major genera of bacteria in the gastrointestinal tract, vagina and mouth of mammals, and are important probiotics. The food industry takes advantage of their beneficial health effects, including regulation of intestinal microbial homeostasis[a] and inhibition of pathogens and pathogenic bacteria that colonize and/or infect the gut mucosa.[b] *Bifidobacterium spp.* also discourage the growth of Gram-negative pathogens in infants.

Lactobacilli are Gram-positive, rod-shaped "good" bacteria that are found as single cells or chains in the flora (i.e. collections of bacterial species) of the mouth and the vagina. Certain *Lactobacillus* species are involved in the production of yogurt, sour cream and buttermilk and many bacteria within this species are the principal components of probiotics formulations.

Pathogenic ("Bad") Gram-positive bacteria

Streptococci are spherical bacteria that occur as chains with some streptococcal species being aerobic and others are anaerobic (these terms are explained below). Although there are harmless

---

[a] The bacterial balance within the intestines

[b] Gomes AMP, Malcata FX. *Bifidobacterium* spp. and *Lactobacillus acidophilus*: biological, biochemical, technological and therapeutical properties relevant for use as probiotics. Trends in Food Science & Technology (1999) 10 (4-5) 139-157.

streptococcal species involved in the production of yogurt, buttermilk and cheese, others are decidedly pathogenic. These include *Streptococcus pneumoniae,* the cause of secondary bacterial pneumonias, and *Streptococcus pyogenes,* the causative agent of "strep throat".

Staphylococci occur in clusters and are normally present on the skin and in mucous membranes. Certain species of staphylococci are involved in skin pathologies such as boils, abscesses and carbuncles. *Staphylococcus aureus* is involved in such pathologies as food poisoning, toxic shock syndrome, pneumonia and staphylococcal meningitis.

Bacillus and *Clostridium* species are rod-shaped bacteria that produce highly resistant spores which are found in the soil, air and within the body. Most species of *Bacillus* grow aerobically, and the deadliest species is *Bacillus anthracis,* the cause of anthrax. In contrast, *Clostridium* species grow anaerobically, and different species cause such pathological conditions as tetanus, botulism and gas gangrene, as mentioned in Chapter 8.

Actinomyces species are Gram-positive rods that are anaerobic, with one species, *A. bovis,* causing the infection known as "lumpy jaw" that occurs in humans and cattle. Although *A. bovis* is a <u>bacterium</u> that resides in the mouths of healthy humans and animals, lumpy jaw is an infection of the jawbone due to these bacteria entering small wounds in the mouth such as those caused by tooth eruption or abrasions by coarse foodstuffs.

Aerobic and anaerobic bacteria

Bacteria are also classified into two broad groups - aerobic and anaerobic - based on their requirement of oxygen. Anaerobic bacteria (anaerobes) are able to survive without the presence of oxygen whereas aerobic bacteria (aerobes) grow and multiply only in the presence of oxygen.

Anaerobic bacteria

There are three types of anaerobic bacteria. These are *obligate* anaerobes which cannot survive in the presence of oxygen, *aerotolerant* anaerobes which do not use oxygen for growth but can tolerate its presence, and *facultative* anaerobes, that can grow without oxygen but can use oxygen if it is present. Some anaerobic bacteria are pathogenic and can cause sinus infections, colds, fevers, ear infections and sexually transmitted diseases like syphilis, gonorrhea and chlamydia. A common facultative (i.e. can live with or without oxygen) anaerobe is *E. coli (Escherichia Coli)* which is present in the intestinal tract of human beings, mammals and birds but which can cause acute respiratory problems, diarrhea and urinary tract infections. *Staphylococcus* is a genus of facultative anaerobe that are found on the mucous membranes and human skin. One species, *Staphylococcus aureus*, can cause ordinary skin infections like boils and acne as well as potentially fatal infections like meningitis, pneumonia and toxic shock syndrome.

Anaerobic bacterial infections can be difficult to treat and often require extended antibiotic treatment for recalcitrant infections.

Aerobic bacteria (aerobes)

Microorganisms that require oxygen for cellular respiration, that is, they need oxygen to survive, grow and reproduce are known as obligate aerobic bacteria although, as mentioned above, facultative bacteria (such as *E. coli and Staphylococcus spp.*) can behave both aerobically and anaerobically, depending on the prevailing conditions. There are also microaerophilic bacteria which require oxygen for their survival but only at a very low concentration. An example of a microaerophilic bacterium is *Helicobacter pylori (H. pylori),* which is present in with patients that suffer from chronic gastritis and gastric ulcers although over 80% of individuals infected with the bacterium are asymptomatic (i.e. have no symptoms). Interestingly, *H. pylori* may play an important role in the natural functioning of the gastro-intestinal system.

The major roles of aerobic bacteria within the body are in the recycling of nutrients, decomposing waste products and assisting in absorption of nutrients by plants.

Antibiotics

As noted above, there are vast numbers of pathogenic bacteria which cause disease although the body is programmed to destroy invasive bacteria through the immune system. In situations where the immune system of the patient is compromised or cannot otherwise deal with bacterial infections, these pathogens customarily are dealt with by antimicrobials such as antibiotics. The latter enhance or augment the immune system's ability to deal with pathogens either by killing bacteria (bactericidal action) or slowing their growth by inhibiting their multiplication (bacteriostatic action).

The first antibiotic was penicillin, discovered in 1928 by Sir Alexander Fleming, and it ushered in the antibiotic era. Medicine changed forever in the early 1950's, when large scale production of penicillin became possible. The term "antibiotic" originally was applied only to antimicrobials derived from living organisms such as molds, yeasts or other microorganisms. In contrast, "chemotherapeutic agents" are purely synthetic in origin although they have bacteriostatic or bactericidal activity against pathogenic microorganisms. Nowadays, all antimicrobials are known as antibiotics, including naturally-derived, semi-synthetic and wholly synthetic therapeutics. Conventional antibiotics, however, are not effective in nonbacterial infections such as viral or fungal infections and individual antibiotics vary widely in their effectiveness on different species of bacteria.

Antibiotics typically are classified by target specificity. Narrow-spectrum antibiotics are used to treat particular types of microorganisms, e.g. specifically Gram-negative or Gram-positive bacteria, whereas broad-spectrum antibiotics can treat a wider range of bacteria. The effectiveness of an individual antibiotic varies with the type of infection, the infection site and its ability to reach that site through its blood supply. Antibiotic efficacy also depends upon the ability of the bacteria to resist or inactivate the administered antibiotic. Whereas antibiotics are considered to be relatively harmless to the host when used to treat infections, they often have an adverse effect on indigenous bacteria, particularly within the gut.

It has been found over the latter part of the 20th century and now into the 21st Century that the clinical effectiveness of antibiotics is decreasing, in some cases alarmingly so. There are various causes of this problem, including overuse and inappropriate administration of antibiotics as well as mutations within many species of bacteria, so that some bacteria are resistant to all antibiotics. The prevalence of antibiotic resistance is rising, with some 60% of nosocomial (hospital acquired) infections now being antibiotic-resistant. This problem has in part stimulated study of essential oils to treat bacterial infections.

GLOSSARY

<u>Aerosol</u>: a mixture of gas and liquid particles in the form of droplets.

<u>Allergen</u>: an entity or substance that induces an allergic reaction.

<u>Allergic reaction</u>: a reaction caused by the immune system overreacting to an allergen and triggering symptoms that can range from mild to life-threatening.

<u>Alopecia</u>: baldness or loss of hair.

<u>Alopecia areata</u>: loss of body or scalp hair in spots.

<u>Androgenetic alopecia</u>: male pattern baldness.

<u>Aerobic bacteria</u> (aerobes): bacteria that require oxygen to perform cellular respiration and which grow and multiply only in the presence of oxygen.

<u>Anaerobic bacteria</u> (anaerobes): bacteria that can survive without oxygen for their growth and multiplication.

<u>Anecdotal</u>: evidence consisting of reports and observations of, usually unscientific, observers that are not necessarily accurate or reliable because they are based on personal accounts rather than facts or research.

<u>Antibacterial</u>: the action of inhibiting bacterial growth or killing bacteria.

<u>Antibiotic</u>: an agent or substance produced by a microorganism that can inhibit the growth or kill another microorganism.

Antibody: protein substances developed by the body in response to an antigen.

Antigen: substance that induces the formation of antibodies; antibodies provide immunity against the disease-producing agent inducing antibody formation.

Anti-ischemic: drug action that improves blood flow to the heart to protect against a heart attack.

Antimicrobial: the action of inhibiting the growth or killing microorganism, e.g. bacteria

Antioxidant: a molecule that can slow or prevent the oxidation of other molecules and which can terminate chain reactions caused by free radicals formed in oxidation reactions. Antioxidants are often reducing agents such as polyphenols.

Anxiolytic: anxiety-reducing action.

Aromatherapy: therapeutic use of essential oils from plants to improve the quality of life

Aromatherapy massage: combination of massage therapy and aromatherapy using essential oils.

Asymptomatic: a disease is considered asymptomatic if a patient carries that disease or infection but has none of its usual symptoms. Asymptomatic infections are also called subclinical infections.

Atopic dermatitis: inflammation of the skin of unknown etiology characterized by itching and scratching.

Bacteria (plural of bacterium): single-celled microscopic organisms that live in water, soil, organic matter or animal bodies and plants; significant as pathogens or their chemical effects.

Bactericidal: the action of a drug that destroys bacteria.

Bacteriostatic: the action of a drug that inhibits bacterial growth.

Bacteriotherapy: (also known as Bacterioprophylaxis) is commonly referred to as replacement therapy and is the application of probiotics to competitively reduce levels of pathogenic bacteria.

Bioactivity: the term applied when a material or agent interacts with or has an effect on any cell tissue in the human body.

<u>Bifidobacteria</u>: Gram-positive anaerobic bacteria found in the gastrointestinal tract and vagina and one of the major genera of bacteria that reside in the colon. Before the 1960s, *Bifidobacterium* species were collectively referred to as "*Lactobacillus bifidus*".

<u>Biosystem</u>: comprehensive term for the human body and its various component organs and systems.

<u>CAM</u>: Complementary or alternative medicine therapeutic modalities to treat disease and includes aromatherapy, massage therapy and chiropractic among other approaches (see Table 4.1).

<u>Carotenoids</u>: or tetraterpenoids, are organic pigments that are produced by plants and algae.

<u>Catechins</u>: polyphenols present in tea and coffee.

<u>CFU</u> (Colony-forming unit): a measure of the numbers of viable bacterial or fungal species, the results commonly being expressed as CFU/mL (colony-forming units per milliliter) in liquids and CFU/g (colony-forming units per gram) in solids.

<u>Chemotherapy</u>: treatment of disease by the administration of drugs.

<u>Comedic</u>: causes blackheads.

<u>Cutaneous</u>: relating to or affecting the skin.

<u>Cytotoxicity</u>: the ability of certain chemicals or mediator cells to destroy living cells either by inducing necrosis (accidental cell death) or apoptosis (programmed cell death).

<u>Disease</u>: an abnormality of structure or function with an identifiable pathological basis and has a recognizable set of clinical signs and/or a condition that is identifiable by chemical, hematological, microbiological, biophysical or immunological means.

<u>Electroencephalogram (EEG)</u>: electrophysiological monitoring of the electrical activity of the brain by measuring voltage fluctuations due to ionic current within the neurons of the brain.

<u>Embrocation</u>: moistening and massage lotion for the skin.

<u>Emolient</u>: agent that has a soft and soothing action on the skin.

<u>Endemic disease</u>: a disorder caused by health conditions constantly present within a community; the term commonly applies to an infection transmitted directly or indirectly between humans.

<u>Endogenous</u>: produced or arising within a cell or an organism.

<u>Enfleurage</u>: (also known as maceration) the use of animal fats such as lard and tallow to leach essential oils from the seeds, petals and even whole flowers of the source plant.

<u>Enteric</u>: term for an entity relating to, or affecting, the intestines

<u>Enzyme</u>: organic catalyst produced by living cells; enzymes are complex proteins that catalyze chemical changes in other substances without undergoing change themselves. Many enzymes have the suffix *ase* indicating the substance they act upon, e.g. acetylcholinesterase breaks down acetylcholine.

<u>Episiotomy</u>: Incision of the perineum at the end of the 2nd stage of labor to avoid laceration and facilitate delivery.

<u>ESCF</u>: European Scientific Committee on Food.

<u>Essential oils (EOs)</u>: (also known as volatile oils) aromatic oily liquids obtained from plant materials (flowers, buds, seeds, leaves, twigs, bark, herbs, wood, fruits and roots).

<u>Extraction</u>: physical or chemical processing method to obtain specific components from plant-based raw materials.

<u>FAO</u>: Food and Agriculture Organization of the United Nations

<u>FDA</u>: U.S. Food and Drug Administration.

<u>FSA</u>: UK Food Standards Agency.

<u>Facultative</u>: the ability of a bacterium to live with or without a specific agent such as oxygen.

<u>Flavonoids</u>: diverse group of phytonutrients (plant chemicals) found in almost all fruits and vegetables, some of the best known being catechins, anthocyanidins and quercetin. Flavonoids have antioxidant and anti-inflammatory health benefits, and together with carotenoids, contribute to the color of fruits and vegetables s.

<u>Flora</u>: collections of bacterial species occurring in or adapted to living in a specific environment.

<u>Fructan</u>: a polymer of fructose molecules. Short chain length fructans are known as fructooligosaccharides, whereas longer chain fructans are termed inulins.

<u>Fungicide</u>: agent that acts against fungi and fungal infections.

Gas Chromatography: an analytical technique in which chemical compounds are vaporized and then separated based on their molecular weight prior to analysis by another technique such as mass spectrometry.

(Gas) Gangrene: potentially fatal infection of a wound caused by bacterial toxins such as *Clostridium perfringens*. Manifests as tissue death and subcutaneous swelling and gas.

Gastrointestinal (GI) tract: The digestive tract, gut or alimentary canal is an organ system in humans and animals that takes in food, digests it to extract and absorb nutrients, and then expels residual matter as feces and urine.

Genus: a group of closely-related species.

Glycogen: large, branched polymer of linked glucose residues (portions of larger molecules) that is the principal way of storing glucose in animal cells.

Homeostasis: bacterial balance within the intestines and elsewhere in the body.

Hydrophilic: literally "water-loving" or miscible with water.

Hydrophobic: water-repelling or immiscible with water.

In Vitro: Laboratory-based scientific studies on biological materials.

In Vivo: Scientific studies performed using animals or humans.

Indigenous: native to a country, region or the human biosystem.

Lactobacillus: genus of Gram-positive, facultative anaerobic bacteria; major part of the lactic acid bacteria group that is important to the microbiota in numerous body sites.

Lactone: a cyclic ester, usually formed by reaction of a carboxylic acid group with a hydroxyl group or halogen atom in the same molecule.

Lactose: a disaccharide sugar formed from galactose and glucose that makes up 2~8% of milk by weight, although the actual content varies between species and individuals.

Leukopenia: decrease in the number of white blood cells (leukocytes) in the blood which can place individuals at increased risk of infection.

Ligand: an entity that binds to a complex central ion or to a substrate.

Lipoprotein: conjugated (coupled together) proteins consisting of simple proteins combined with lipids (fats), e.g. cholesterol and triglycerides.

Literature: the term applied to published reports and reviews of scientific studies in scientific/professional journals and books.

Mass spectrometry: an analytical technique in which chemical compounds are ionized to generate charged molecules that are then measured for their charge-to-mass ratio.

Microbiota: community of microorganisms that include bacteria, fungi and viruses that co-exist in plants and animals, are crucial for immunologic, hormonal and metabolic homeostasis of the host.

Minimum inhibitory concentration (MIC): of an antibacterial is the maximum dilution of that drug that will still inhibit the growth of a test microorganism.

Morbid: affected by disease; related to or characteristic of disease.

Morbidity: state of being diseased or the number of persons affected by a disease within a specific population.

Naturopathy: therapeutic system that uses natural forces (light, heat, air, water and massage) for patient treatment rather than drugs.

Nebulizer: device that uses oxygen, compressed air or ultrasonic vibrations to break up liquids and solutions into small aerosol droplets that are emitted into the air for inhalation. Also known as a diffuser or vaporizer.

Nitric oxide (NO): an important messenger molecule involved in many physiological (and pathological) processes. It is a signaling molecule often involved in transmitting information between cells by interacting with receptors in another cell to trigger a response.

Nosocomial: hospital acquired, as in nosocomial infections.

Olfactory: relating to the sense of smell.

Oligo: scientific term for a few.

Oligodynamic effect: toxic effect of metal-ions on living cells and microorganisms, even in relatively low concentrations. This antimicrobial effect is shown by ions of many metals, including aluminum, bismuth, copper, gold, iron, lead, mercury, silver and zinc. Both Gram-positive and Gram-negative bacteria may be affected by the oligodynamic effect although they can develop a heavy-metal resistance.

Oligofructose: a subgroup of inulin, consisting of polymers with up to 10 polymer units; stimulates intestinal bifidobacteria.

Oligosaccharide: (also known as compound sugar) a short chain of sugar molecules consisting of 2-8 monosaccharide units linked by glycoside bonds..

Organelle: part of a cell that performs a definite function.

Oxidation: a chemical reaction in which electrons are transferred from a substance to an oxidizing agent; oxidation reactions can produce free radicals which, in turn, can initiate chain reactions that damage cells.

pH: the pH of an aqueous solution is a measure of its acidity or basicity (alkalinity). Pure water is neutral, with a pH close to 7.0, whereas solutions with a pH less than 7 (pH < 7.0) are acidic and those with a pH greater than 7 (pH > 7.0) are basic or alkaline.

Pathogenic: disease-causing.

Pathogenicity: propensity for causing disease.

Pathology: branch of medicine concerned with structural and functional changes within the body caused by disease.

Perineum: connective tissue sheath surrounding nerve fibers.

Phytomedicine: the term for the preventive and therapeutic use of essential oils.

Plasma: liquid part of the lymph and blood.

Polyphenols: a group of chemical substances, commonly antioxidants, found in plants which contain two or more phenol units per molecule; they are divided into the hydrolyzable tannins (e.g. tannic acid) and other sugars, and phenylpropanoids, such as lignins, flavonoids, and condensed tannins.

Polysaccharide: name given to any member of a class of relatively complex, high-molecular weight carbohydrates consisting of long-chains of many monosaccharides (sugars) joined together. Well-known polysaccharides include starch, glycogen, cellulose and chitin.

Prebiotic: selectively fermented food ingredient that beneficially affects the host through specific stimulation of the growth and/or activity of one or more bacteria in the colon.

Probiotic: foodstuff containing a live microbiological culture

Pyrogenetic: causing a fever.

QOL: quality of life.

Reduction: a chemical reaction in which electrons are transferred to a substance by a reducing agent.

Ribonucleic acid (RNA): nucleic acid found in certain cell components and has an important role in synthesizing reactions within cells.

Ruminants: mammals that acquire nutrients from plants through microbial fermentation in a specialized stomach prior to digestion.

Saccharide: scientific term for a sugar.

Species: the largest group of organisms that can interbreed to produce a fertile offspring.

Sucrose: is a disaccharide produced by the condensation of glucose and fructose. Sucrose, commonly known as table sugar, is formed by plants but not by other organisms.

Synbiotic: combination of a prebiotic and probiotic in a single product.

Systolic: pertaining to the systole or contraction of the heart when blood is forced through the circulatory system. Systolic pressure is the upper number in blood pressure measurements.

Tannic acid: polyphenol comprising glucose esters of gallic acid.

Taxonomy: The branch of science dealing with the categorization of organisms into separate groups based on the presence and absence of certain characteristics.

Telemores: the DNA sequences at the end of chromosomes, i.e. the "end filler" of human DNA strands. Telemores shorten with aging and when consumed, the cell is destroyed. Some scientists believe that telomeres, and telomerase the enzyme which controls the lengthening/shortening of telomeres on human DNA, are key to aging and cancer.

<u>Theaflavin</u>: antioxidant polyphenols formed from catechins in tea leaves during the enzymatic oxidation (or fermentation) of the leaves during preparation of black tea.

<u>Theanine</u>: an amino acid commonly found in tea.

<u>Theobromine</u>: an alkaloid of the cacao plant, found in chocolate and in many chocolate-free foods made from theobromine sources including the leaves of the tea plant; it has a similar, but lesser, effect to caffeine.

<u>Trichologist</u>: a hair and scalp treatment specialist.

<u>Urticaria</u>: allergic reaction marked by skin rash, e.g. nettle rash and hives.

<u>Viricide</u>: agent or drug that acts on viruses.

<u>WHO</u>: The World Health Organization

<u>Xanthine</u>: a purine base found in most body tissues and fluids; mild stimulants such as caffeine and theobromine are derived from xanthine.

ABOUT THE AUTHOR

Dr. J. Anthony von Fraunhofer is Professor Emeritus, Health Sciences Center, University of Maryland in Baltimore, Maryland. He studied at Sir John Cass College, University of London where he was awarded a BSc degree with honors in chemistry and then went on to gain his MSc and PhD degrees. He has Chartered Scientist, Chartered Chemist and Chartered Engineer designations from the United Kingdom Science Council. He holds Fellowships in the Academy of Dental Materials, ASM International, the Institute of Corrosion and the Royal Society of Chemistry.

He has written over 400 scientific papers, 17 books, and contributed chapters to 14 multi-author monographs. He has made over 140 research presentations at National/International meetings and lectured and presented courses in the United States, the United Kingdom, Continental Europe, North Africa and the Middle East. His fields of interest and active research efforts include the physical and mechanical properties of biomaterials; dental cutting; wound closure devices, wound healing and the degradation of materials in the biosystem. He also holds a number of patents in the field of biomaterials science.

BIBLIOGRAPHY

[1] Stewart, D. *The chemistry of essential oils made simple.* Care Publications. Marble Hill, MO. (2016).

[2] Wildwood, C. *The Encyclopedia of Aromatherapy.* Healing Arts Press, Rochester, VT (1996).

[3] Davies, E. Smarter smells. Chemistry World (2016) 13: 56-59.

[4] Ritter, S. K. C&EN (2017) 95 (11) 23-25.

[5] Tigrine-Kordjani N. B.Y. Meklati, B. Y. and Chemat, F .Microwave 'dry' distillation as an useful tool for extraction of edible essential oils. International Journal of Aromatherapy (2006) 16: 141-147.

[6] Lucchesi, M. E., Chemat, F. and Smadja, J. Solvent-free microwave extraction of essential oil from aromatic herbs: comparison with conventional hydro-distillation. Journal of Chromatography A (2004) 1043: 323–327.

[7] Golmakani M-T, Rezaei K. Comparison of microwave-assisted hydrodistillation with the traditional hydrodistillation method in the extraction of essential oils from *Thymus vulgaris* L. Food Chemistry (2008) 109: 925–930.

[8] Traditional Medicine Definitions. World Health Organization. (2008)

[9] von Fraunhofer J. A. *Vitamins, Minerals and Spices.* (2013). CreateSpace, Seattle, WA.

[10] Khanna R, MacDonald JK, Levesque BG. Peppermint oil for the treatment of irritable bowel syndrome: a systematic review and meta-analysis. J Clin Gastroenterol (2014) 48(6):505-12.

[11] Pittler MH, Ernst E. Peppermint oil for irritable bowel syndrome: a systematic review and meta-analysis. Am J Gastroenterol. (1998) 93(7):1131-5.

[12] May B, Kuntz HD, Kieser M, Köhler S. Efficacy of a fixed peppermint oil/caraway oil combination in non-ulcer dyspepsia. Arzneimittelforschung. (1996) 46(12):1149-53.

[13] Micklefield GH, Greving I, May B. Effects of peppermint oil and caraway oil on gastroduodenal motility. Phytother Res. (2000) 14(1):20-3.

[14] Haber SL, El-Ibiary SY. Peppermint oil for treatment of irritable bowel syndrome. Am J Health Syst Pharm. (2016) 73(2):22, 24, 26.

[15] Chadwick M, Trewin H, Gawthrop F, Wagstaff C. Sesquiterpenoid Lactones: Benefits to Plants and People. Int. J. Mol. Sci. (2013) 14(6), 12780-12805.

[16] Dimas K, Kokkinopoulos D, Demetzos C, et al. The effect of sclareol on

growth and cell cycle progression of human leukemic cell lines. Leuk Res (1999) 23(3):217-34.

[17] Sylvestre M, Pichette A, Longtin A, et al. Essential oil analysis and anticancer activity of leaf essential oil of Croton flavens L. from Guadeloupe. J Ethnopharmacol. (2006) 103:99–102.

[18] Frank MB, Yang Q, Osban J, et al. Frankincense oil derived from Boswellia carteri induces tumor cell specific cytotoxicity. BMC Complementary and Alternative Medicine (2009) 9: 6.

[19] Su S, Wang T, Ting Chen T, et al. Cytotoxicity activity of extracts and compounds from Commiphora myrrha resin against human gynecologic cancer cells. Journal of Medicinal Plants Research (2011) 5(8): 1382-1389.

[20] Sharma PR, Mondhe DM, Muthiah S, et al. Anticancer activity of an essential oil from Cymbopogon flexuosus. Chem Biol Interact (2009) 179(2-3):160-8.

[21] Bidinotto LT, Costa CA, Costa M, et al. Modifying effects of lemongrass essential oil on specific tissue response to the carcinogen N-methyl-N-nitrosurea in female BALB/c mice. J Med Food (2012) 15(2):161-8.

[22] Wang XL, Kong F, Shen T, et al. Sesquiterpenoids from myrrh inhibit androgen receptor expression and function in human prostate cancer cells. Acta Pharmacol Sin (2011) 32(3):338-44.

[23] Salmani KKA. Frankincense as a Potentially Novel Therapeutic Agent in Ovarian Cancer: Conference Paper presented at the 27th Lorne Cancer Conference 2015, At Mantra Lorne, Lorne, Victoria, Australia.

[24] Wang L, Hong-Sheng He, Hua-Long Yu, et al. Sclareol, a plant diterpene, exhibits potent antiproliferative effects via the induction of apoptosis and mitochondrial membrane potential loss in osteosarcoma cancer cells. Molecular Medicine Reports (2015) 11(6):4273.

[25] Chen Y, Zhou C, Ge Z, et al. Composition and potential anticancer activities of essential oils obtained from myrrh and frankincense. Oncol. Lett. (2013) 6(4): 1140–1146.

[26] Cetin B, Ozer H, Cakir A, Polat T. et al. Antimicrobial activities of essential oil and hexane extract of Florence fennel [Foeniculum vulgare var. azoricum (Mill.) Thell] against foodborne microorganisms. J Med Food (2010) 13(1):196-204.

[27] Kanamakar SS., Khare RH., Ojha S, Kundu K. and Kundu S. Development of Probiotic Candidate in Combination with Essential Oils from Medicinal Plant and Their Effect on Enteric Pathogens: A Review. Gastroenterology Research and Practice (2012), Article ID 457150, 6 pp.

[28] von Fraunhofer J.A. *Prebiotics and Probiotics*. Kindle/CreateSpace, Seattle, WA. (2012).

[29]Bibel DL. Bacterial interference, bacteriotherapy and bacterioprophylaxis. In: *Bacterial interference* (ed. R. Aly and H. R. Shinefield), CRC Press (1982), 1-12.

[30] Elmer GW, Surawicz CM, McFarland LV. Biotherapeutic agents. A neglected modality for the treatment and prevention of selected intestinal and vaginal infections. J Am Med Assoc (1996) 275:870-6.

[31] Tagg JR, Dierksen KP. Bacterial replacement therapy: adapting "germ warfare" to infection prevention. Trends Biotechnol (2003) 21: 217-233.

[32] Tisserand, RB. *Gattefossé's Aromatherapy*. C. W. Daniel Co. Ltd., Saffron Walden, U.K. (1995).

[33] Tisserand, R. *Aromatherapy: To Heal and Tend the Body*. Lotus Press, Silver Lake, WI (1988).

[34] Valnet, J. *The Practice of Aromatherapy*. Healing Arts Press, Randolph, VT (1990).

[35] Buchbauer G, Jirovetz L, Jäger W, et al.: Fragrance compounds and essential oils with sedative effects upon inhalation. J Pharm Sci (1993) 82: 660-4.

[36] Lis-Balchin M. Essential oils and 'aromatherapy': their modern role in healing. J Roy Soc Health (1997) 117(5):324-9.

[37] West B. The essence of aromatherapy. Elder Care (1993) 5(4):24-5.

[38] Cooke B, Ernst E. Aromatherapy: a systematic review. Br J Gen Pract. (2000) 50(455):493-6.

[39] Ades TB, ed. (2009). "Aromatherapy". American Cancer Society Complete Guide to Complementary and Alternative Cancer Therapies (2nd ed.). American Cancer Society. pp. 57–60.

[40] Conrad P, Adams C. The effects of clinical aromatherapy for anxiety and depression in the high risk postpartum woman - a pilot study. Complement Ther Clin Pract. (2012) 18(3):164-8.

[41] Hines, Sonia; Steels, Elizabeth; Chang, Anne; Gibbons, Kristen (2012-04-18). Aromatherapy for treatment of postoperative nausea and vomiting. Cochrane Database of Systematic Reviews. John Wiley & Sons. NJ. (2012)

[42] Sánchez-Vidaña DI, Ngai SP, He W, et al. The Effectiveness of Aromatherapy for Depressive Symptoms: A Systematic Review. Evid Based Complement Alternat Med. (2017) 5869315. Epub 2017 Jan 4

[43] Worwood VA: *Aromatherapy for the Healthy Child: More Than 300 Natural, Non-Toxic, and Fragrant Essential Oil Blends*. New World Library, Novato, CA. (2000).

44 Pibiri M-C., Goel, A, Vahekeni, N., C.-A. Roulet, C-A. Indoor air purification and ventilation systems sanitation with essential oils. International Journal of Aromatherapy (2006) 16: 149-153.

45 Kuriyama, H., Watanabe, S., Nakaya, T., et al. Immunological and Psychological Benefits of Aromatherapy Massage. Evidence-Based Complementary and Alternative Medicine (2005) 2 (2): 179.

46 Butje A, Repede E, Shattell MMJ. Healing scents: an overview of clinical aromatherapy for emotional distress. Psychosoc Nurs Ment Health Serv. (2008) 46(10):46-52.

47 Dodd GH: The molecular dimension in perfumery. In: Van Toller S, Dodd GH, eds.: Perfumery: The Psychology and Biology of Fragrance.: Chapman and Hall, New York, NY (1988), pp 19-46.

48 Proksch E, Brandner JM, Jensen JM "The skin: an indispensable barrier". Exp Dermatol. (2008). 17: 1063–72.

49 Madison KC. Barrier function of the skin: "la raison d'être" of the epidermis. *J Invest Dermatol. (2003) 121: 231–41*

50 Cavalca Cortelli S, Cavallini F, Regueira Alves MF, et al. Clinical and microbiological effects of an essential-oil-containing mouth rinse applied in the "one-stage full-mouth disinfection" protocol--a randomized double-blinded preliminary study. Clin Oral Investig. (2009) 13(2):189-94.

51 Cosyn J, Princen K, Miremadi R,et al. A double-blind randomized placebo-controlled study on the clinical and microbial effects of an essential oil mouth rinse used by patients in supportive periodontal care. Int J Dent Hyg. (2013) 11(1):53-61.

52 Javed F, Al-Hezaimi K, Romanos GE. Role of dentifrices with essential oil formulations in periodontal healing. Am J Med Sci. (2012) 343(5):411-7.

53 Altaei DT. Topical lavender oil for the treatment of recurrent aphthous ulceration. Am J Dent. (2012) 25(1):39-43.

54 Hur MH, Han SH. Clinical trial of aromatherapy on postpartum mother's perineal healing. Taehan Kanho Hakhoe Chi (2004) 34:53-62.

55 Sheikhan F, Jahdi F, Khoei EM, et al. Episiotomy pain relief: Use of Lavender oil essence in primiparous Iranian women. Complement Ther Clin Pract. (2012) 18(1):66-70.

56 Marzouk T, Barakat R, Ragab A, et al. Lavender-thymol as a new topical aromatherapy preparation for episiotomy: A randomised clinical trial. J Obstet Gynaecol. (2015) 35:472-5.

57 Cash TF, Price VH, Savin RC. Psychological effects of androgenetic alopecia on women: comparisons with balding men and with female control subjects. J Am Acad Dematol (1993) 29:568–575.

[58] Hadshiew IM, Foitzik K, Arck PC, Paus R. Burden of hair loss: stress and the underestimated psychosocial impact of telogen effluvium and androgenetic alopecia. J Invest Dermatol (2004) 123:455–457.

[59] Stough D., Stenn K., Haber R., et al. Psychological effect, pathophysiology, and management of androgenetic alopecia in men. *Mayo Clin. Proc.* (2005) 80:1316–1322

[60] Lee BH, Lee JS and Kim YC. Hair Growth-Promoting Effects of Lavender Oil in C57BL/6 Mice. Toxicol Res (2016) 32(2): 103–108.

[61] Panahi Y, Taghizadeh M, Marzony ET, Sahebkar A. Rosemary oil vs minoxidil 2% for the treatment of androgenetic alopecia: a randomized comparative trial. Skinmed. (2015) 13(1):15-21.

[62] Hay IC, Jamieson M, Ormerod AD. Randomized trial of aromatherapy. Successful treatment for alopecia areata. Arch Dermatol (1998)134(11):1349-52.

[63] Young Oh J, Min Ah Park, M, and Young Chul Kim, Y. Peppermint Oil Promotes Hair Growth without Toxic Signs. Toxicol. Res. (2014) 30(4): 297–304.

[64] Chaisripipat W, Lourith N, Kanlayavattanakul M. Anti-dandruff Hair Tonic Containing Lemongrass (Cymbopogon flexuosus) Oil. Forsch Komplementmed (2015) 22(4):226-9.

[65] Salvo SG. *Massage Therapy: Principles and Practice*, 5th Edition. Saunders, St Lois MO (2016).

[66] Fritz S. *Mosby's Fundamentals of Therapeutic Massage*, 6th Edition Elsevier, St. Louis, MO. (2017).

[67] Beck M F. *Theory and Practice of Therapeutic Massage* 5th Edition, Milady Inc., Boston, MA (2017).

[68] Clarke TC, Nahin, RL, Barnes PM, et al. Use of Complementary Health Approaches for Musculoskeletal Pain Disorders Among Adults: United States, 2012. National Health Statistics Reports Number 98. National Center for Health Statistics, Washington, D.C. (2016).

[69] Cherkin DC, Sherman KJ, Kahn J, et al. A comparison of the effects of 2 types of massage and usual care on chronic low back pain: a randomized, controlled trial. Annals of Internal Medicine (2011) 155:1–9.

[70] Furlan AD, Imamura M, Dryden T, et al. Massage for low-back pain. Cochrane Database of Systematic Reviews (2008) No. 4:CD001929.

[71] Perlman AI, Ali A, Njike VY, et al. Massage therapy for osteoarthritis of the knee: a randomized dose-finding trial. PLoS One (2012) 7(2): e30248.

[72] Sherman KJ, Ludman EJ, Cook AJ, et al. Effectiveness of therapeutic massage for generalized anxiety disorder: a randomized controlled trial. Depression and Anxiety (2010) 27: 441–450.

[73] Kalichman, L. Massage therapy for fibromyalgia symptoms. Rheumatology International (2010) 30:1151–1157.

[74] Bennett C, Underdown A, Barlow J. Massage for promoting mental and physical health in typically developing infants under the age of six months. Cochrane Database of Systematic Review. (2013) No. 4:CD005038.

[75] Lee MS, Kim JI, Ernst E. Massage therapy for children with autism spectrum disorders: a systematic review. Journal of Clinical Psychiatry (2011) 72:406–411.

[76] Hondras MA, Linde K., Jones AP. Manual therapy for asthma. Cochrane Database of Systematic Reviews (2006).

[77] Hillier SL, Louw Q, Morris L, et al. Massage therapy for people with HIV/AIDS. Cochrane Database of Systematic Reviews (2010) No. 1: CD007502.

[78] Chen TH, Tung TH, Chen PS, et al. The Clinical Effects of Aromatherapy Massage on Reducing Pain for the Cancer Patients: Meta-Analysis of Randomized Controlled Trials. Evid. Based Complement. Alternat. Med. (2016) 9147974. Epub 2016 Jan 14.

[79] Ein-Soon S, Kyung-Hwa S, Sun-Hee L, et al. Massage with or without aromatherapy for symptom relief in people with cancer. Cochrane Database of Systematic Reviews (2016) June.

[80] Prabuseenivasan, S., Jayakumar, M. and Ignacimuthu, S. *In vitro* antibacterial activity of some plant essential oils. BMC Complement Altern Med (2006) 6: 39-50.

[81] Tisserand, RB. *Gattefossé's Aromatherapy*. C. W. Daniel Co. Ltd., Saffron Walden, U.K. (1995).

[82] Tisserand, R. *Aromatherapy: To Heal and Tend the Body*. Lotus Press, Silver Lake, WI (1988).

[83] Valnet, J. *The Practice of Aromatherapy*. Healing Arts Press, Randolph, VT (1990).

[84] Cavanagh HM, Wilkinson JM. Biological activities of lavender essential oil. Phytother. Res. (2002) 16:301–308.

[85] Gattefossé RM. « Emplois des huiles essentielles comme bactéricides » *La Parfumerie Moderne*, 1932, 533

[86] Gattefossé RM. « Rôle antiseptique de la lavande » *La Parfumerie Moderne* (1932) 26 : 543-553.

[87] Valnet J. *L'Aromathérapie* ou *Aromathérapie, Traitement des maladies par les essences des plantes*, Paris, éd. Le Livre de Poche N°7885, Paris, (1964).

[88] Valnet J, Duraffourd Ch, Lapraz J-Cl., *Une médecine nouvelle. Phytothérapie et aromathérapie - comment guérir les maladies infectieuses par les plantes*, éd. Presses de la Renaissance, Paris, France. (1978).

[89] Valnet J. *The Practice of Aromatherapy*. Beekman Books Inc; 7th edition. Beekman Books, Inc., Wappingers Falls, New York. (1990).

[90] Burt SA. Essential oils: their antibacterial properties and potential applications in foods: a review. Inter J Food Microbiol (2004) 94:223–253.

[91] Faid M, Bakhy K, Anchad M, Tantaoui-Elaraki A, Almond paste: Physicochemical and microbiological characterizations and preservation with sorbic acid and cinnamon. J Food Prod (1995) 58:547–550.

[92] Chadwick M, Trewin H, Gawthrop F, Wagstaff C.. Sesquiterpenoids Lactones: Benefits to Plants and People. Int. J. Mol. Sci. (2013) 14(6), 12780-12805.

[93] Haffor AS. Effect of myrrh (Commiphora molmol) on leukocyte levels before and during healing from gastric ulcer or skin injury. J Immunotoxicol (2010) 7(1):68-75.

[94] Nomicos EYH. Myrrh: medical marvel or myth of the Magi? Holistic Nursing Practice (2007) 21(6):308.

[95] Sienkiewicz M, Łysakowska M, Pastuszka M, et al. The potential of use basil and rosemary essential oils as effective antibacterial agents. Molecules (2013) 18(8): 9334-51.

[96] Wanner J, Schmidt E, Bail S, et al. Chemical composition and antibacterial activity of selected essential oils and some of their main compounds. Nat. Prod. Commun. (2010) 5(9):1359-64.

[97] Sienkiewicz M, Poznańska-Kurowska, K. Kaszuba, A, et al. The antibacterial activity of geranium oil against Gram-negative bacteria isolated from difficult-to-heal wounds. Burns (2014) 40:1046-51.

[98] Forbes MA, Schmid MM. Use of OTC essential oils to clear plantar warts. Nurse Pract (2006) 31(3):53-55, 57.

[99] Sienkiewicz M, Głowacka A, Kowalczyk E, et al. The biological activities of cinnamon, geranium and lavender essential oils. Molecules. (2014) 19: 20929-40.

[100] Sienkiewicz M, Łysakowska M, Denys P, et al. The antimicrobial activity of thyme essential oil against multidrug resistant clinical bacterial strains. Microb Drug Resist. (2012) 18:137-48.

[101] Knezevic P, Aleksic V, Simin N, et al. Antimicrobial activity of Eucalyptus camaldulensis essential oils and their interactions with conventional antimicrobial agents against multi-drug resistant Acinetobacter baumannii. J Ethnopharmacol. (2016) 178:125-36.

[102] National Institute for Health and Care Excellence. "Fungal nail infection" *(Clinical Knowledge Summary),* London, UK. *2014.*

[103] National Institute for Health and Care Excellence. "Fungal skin infection - foot" *(Clinical Knowledge Summary),* London, UK, 2014.

[104] de Rapper S, Van Vuuren SF, Kamatou GP, et al. The additive and synergistic antimicrobial effects of select frankincense and myrrh oils--a combination from the pharaonic pharmacopoeia. Lett. Appl. Microbiol. (2012) 54(4):352-8.

[105] Thomsen PS, Jensen TM, Hammer KA, et al. Survey of the antimicrobial activity of commercially available Australian tea tree (Melaleuca alternifolia) essential oil products in vitro. J Altern Complement Med. (2011) 17(9):835-41.

[106] Pazyar N, Yaghoobi R, Bagherani N, Kazerouni A. A review of applications of tea tree oil in dermatology. Int J Dermatol. (2013) 52(7):784-90.

[107] Li WR, Li HL, Shi QS, et al. The dynamics and mechanism of the antimicrobial activity of tea tree oil against bacteria and fungi. Appl. Microbiol. Biotechnol. (2016) 100(20):8865-75.

[108] Thomas J, Carson CF, Peterson GM, et al. Therapeutic Potential of Tea Tree Oil for Scabies. Am. J. Trop. Med. Hyg.(2016) 94(2):258-66.

[109] Eisenhower C, Farrington EA. Advancements in the Treatment of Head Lice in Pediatrics. Journal of Pediatric Health Car. (2012) 26: 451–61.

[110] Chin KB, Cordell B. The effect of tea tree oil (Melaleuca alternifolia) on wound healing using a dressing model. J Altern. Complement. Med. (2013) 19(12):942-5.

[111] Donoyama, N. and Ichiman, Y. Which essential oil is better for hygienic massage practice? Int. J. Aromatherapy (2006) 16:175–179.

[112] Keane FM, Smith HR, White IR, Rycroft RJ. Occupational allergic contact dermatitis in two aromatherapists. Contact Dermatitis (2000) 43(1):49-51.

[113] Bleasel N, Tate B, Rademaker M. Allergic contact dermatitis following exposure to essential oils. Australas J Dermatol (2002) 43(3):211-3.

[114] Boonchai W, Iamtharachai P, Sunthonpalin P. Occupational allergic contact dermatitis from essential oils in aromatherapists. Contact Dermatitis (2007) 56(3):181-2.

[115] Craig WJ. Health-promoting properties of common herbs. Am. J. Clin. Nutr. (1999) 70(3 Suppl):491S-499S.

[116] Kalemba D, Kunicka A. Antibacterial and antifungal properties of essential oils. Curr. Med. Chem. (2003) 10(10):813-29.

117 Wanner J, Schmidt E, Bail S, et al. Chemical composition and antibacterial activity of selected essential oils and some of their main compounds. Nat Prod Commun. (2010) 5(9):1359-64.

118 Khallouki F, Younos C, Soulimani R, et al.. Consumption of argan oil (Morocco) with its unique profile of fatty acids, tocopherols, squalene, sterols and phenolic compounds should confer valuable cancer chemopreventive effects. Eur. J. Cancer Prev. (2003)12(1):67-75.

119 Monfalouti HE, Guillaume D, Denhez C, et al . Z. Therapeutic potential of argan oil: a review. J. Pharm. Pharmacol. (2010) 62(12):1669-75.

120 Charrouf Z, Guillaume D. Phenols and Polyphenols from Argania spinosa. American Journal of Food Technology (2007) 2 (7): 679.

121 Khallouki, F; Younos, C; Soulimani, R, et al. Consumption of argan oil (Morocco) with its unique profile of fatty acids, tocopherols, squalene, sterols and phenolic compounds should confer valuable cancer chemopreventive effects. European Journal of Cancer Prevention (2003) 12 (1): 67–75.

122 Charrouf Z. Guillaume D. Argan oil: Occurrence, composition and impact on human health. European Journal of Lipid Science and Technology (2008) 110 (7): 632.

123 Charrouf Z, Guillaume D Should the Amazigh Diet (Regular and Moderate Argan-Oil Consumption) have a Beneficial Impact on Human Health?. Crit. Rev. Food Sci. Nutr. (2010) 50): 473–7.

124 Vaughn AR, Clark AK, Sivamani RK, et al. Natural Oils for Skin-Barrier Repair: Ancient Compounds Now Backed by Modern Science. Am. J. Clin. Dermatol. (2017) Jul 13. doi: 10.1007/s40257-017-0301-1. [Epub ahead of print]

125 Busson-Breysse J; Farines M, Soulier J. Jojoba wax: Its esters and some of its minor components. Journal of the American Oil Chemist' Society (1994) 71 (9): 999–1002.

126 Hicks, SC, Siemer, SR. Method of controlling powdery mildew infections of plants using jojoba wax. USP 6,174,920 (2001).

127 Pazyar N, Yaghoobi R, Ghassemi MR, et al. Jojoba in dermatology: a succinct review. G Ital Dermatol Venereol (2013) 148(6):687-91.

128 Reichling J, Schnitzler P, Suschke U, et al. Essential oils of aromatic plants with antibacterial, antifungal, antiviral, and cytotoxic properties--an overview. Forsch. Komplementmed. (2009) 16(2):79-90.

129 Zhu J, Lower-Nedza AD, Hong M, et al. Chemical composition and antimicrobial activity of three essential oils from Curcuma wenyujin. Nat. Prod. Commun. (2013) 8(4):523-6.

130 Zhang L, Yang Z, Chen D, et al. Variation on composition and bioactivity of essential oils of four common Curcuma herbs. Chem. Biodivers. (2017) Aug 10. doi: 10.1002/cbdv.201700280. [Epub ahead of print]

131 Ashour ML, El-Readi M, Youns M, et al. Chemical composition and biological activity of the essential oil obtained from Bupleurum marginatum (Apiaceae). J Pharm. Pharmacol. (2009) 61(8):1079-87.

132 Dahham SS, Hassan LE, Ahamed MB, et al. In vivo toxicity and antitumor activity of essential oils extract from agarwood (Aquilaria crassna). BMC Complement Altern. Med. (2016) 16:236.

133 Dahham SS, Tabana YM, Iqbal MA, et al. The Anticancer, Antioxidant and Antimicrobial Properties of the Sesquiterpene β-Caryophyllene from the Essential Oil of Aquilaria crassna. Molecules. (2015) 20(7):11808-29.

134 Maia JGS, Andrade EHA, Carreira LMM, et al. Essential oils of the Amazon *Guatteria* and *Guatteriopsis* species. Flavor and Fragrance J. (2005) 20: 478–480.

135 Costa EV, Teixeira SD, Marques FA, et al. Chemical composition and antimicrobial activity of the essential oils of the Amazon Guatteriopsis species. Phytochemistry (2008) 69(9):1895-9.

136 Santos AR, Benghi TGS, Nepel A, et al. In vitro Antiproliferative and Antibacterial Activities of Essential Oils from Four Species of Guatteria. Chem Biodivers. 2017 Jul 18. doi: 10.1002/cbdv.201700097. [Epub ahead of print].

137 de Lima BR, da Silva FM, Soares ER, et al. Chemical composition and antimicrobial activity of the essential oils of Onychopetalum amazonicum R.E.Fr. Nat. Prod. Res. (2016) 30(20):2356-9.

138 Costa EV, Menezes LR, Rocha SL, et al. Antitumor Properties of the leaf essential oil of Zornia brasiliensis. Planta Med. (2015) 81(7):563-7.

139 Khadir A, Sobeh M, Gad HA, et al. Chemical composition and biological activity of the essential oil from Thymus lanceolatus. Z. Naturforsch. C. (2016) 71(5-6):155-63.

140 Cardile V, Russo A, Formisano C, et al. Essential oils of Salvia bracteata and Salvia rubifolia from Lebanon: Chemical composition, antimicrobial activity and inhibitory effect on human melanoma cells. J. Ethnopharmacol. (2009) 126(2):265-72.

141 Stojanović G, Palić I. Antimicrobial and antioxidant activity of Micromeria Bentham species. Curr. Pharm. Des. (2008) 14(29):3196-202.

142 Aleksic V, Knezevic P. Antimicrobial and antioxidative activity of extracts and essential oils of Myrtus communis L Microbiol. Res. (2014) 169(4):240-54.

143 Fraternale D, Bucchini A, Giamperi L, et al. Essential oil composition and antimicrobial activity of Ballota nigra L. ssp foetida. Nat. Prod. Commun. (2009) 4(4):585-8.

144 Craig WJ. Health-promoting properties of common herbs. Am. J. Clin. Nutr. (1999) 70(3 Suppl):491S-499S.

145 Shareef M, Ashraf MA, Sarfraz M. Natural cures for breast cancer treatment. Saudi Pharm. J. (2016) 24(3):233-40.

146 Russo A, Cardile V, Graziano AC, et al. Comparison of essential oil components and in vitro anticancer activity in wild and cultivated Salvia verbenaca. Nat. Prod. Res. (2015) 29(17):1630-40.

147 Fontes JEdoN, Ferraz RPC, Britto ACS, et al. Antitumor Effect of the Essential Oil from Leaves of *Guatteria pogonopus* (Annonaceae). Chemistry and Biodivertisy (2013) 10: 722-729.

[148] Santos AR, Benghi TGS, Nepel A, et al.   In vitro Antiproliferative and Antibacterial Activities of Essential Oils from Four Species of Guatteria. Chem Biodivers. 2017 Jul 18. doi: 10.1002/cbdv.201700097. [Epub ahead of print]

[149] Edris AE. Anti-cancer properties of Nigella spp. essential oils and their major constituents, thymoquinone and beta-elemene. Curr. Clin. Pharmacol. (2009) 4(1):43-6.

[150] Yan R, Yang Y, Zeng Y, et al. Cytotoxicity and antibacterial activity of Lindera strychnifolia essential oils and extracts. J. Ethnopharmacol. (2009) 121(3):451-5.

[151] Nerurkar P, Ray RB. Bitter melon: antagonist to cancer. Pharm. Res. (2010) 27(6):1049-53.

[152] Dandawate PR, Subramaniam D, Padhye SB, et al. Bitter melon: a panacea for inflammation and cancer. Chin. J. Nat. Med. (2016) 14(2):81-100.

[153] Lesgards JF, Baldovini N, Vidal N, et al. Anticancer activities of essential oils constituents and synergy with conventional therapies: a review. Phytother. Res. (2014) 28(10):1423-46.

INDEX

Fermentation	1,9,51,105,120,121
Folk medicine	*See CAM*
Fragrance	1,2,4,7,8,11,12,13,15,16,29,34,88
Frankincense	16,21,31,35,54,55,58,73,74,76
Fragrance	1,2,4,7,8,11,12,13,15,16,29,34,58,73
Fruit juice	11
Fungal infection	19,34,52,55,64,112,116
Gattefossé	25,53,54,58
Glossary	113-121
Gram negative bacteria	106-108
Gram positive bacteria	65,66,67,91,106,108-109
Gram staining	106
Grapefruit	2,11,16,22,30
GRAS	23
Guatteria and Guatteriopsis	65,66
Harvesting	9,61,83,87
Healthcare	29,54,57,92
Herbs	1,20,57,70,86,90,91,116
Herbicide	4,10
HIV	46,47
Hydrodistillation	*See Distillation*
Hydrophobicity	7,117
Hypertension	43
Joint pain	*See Muscle and Joint Pain*
Jojoba oil	60,61-62
Lactone	23,117
Lard	3,12
Lavender oil	1,12,22,38,52,53,91
Lemongrass oil	22,35,39,41,45,53,54
Lindera	63,69
Maceration	12,15,82,85,115
Massage oils	36,44,45
Massage therapy	4,7,20,34,36,37,41,43-49,114,115,118
Melissa (lemon balm)	22,31,35
Menstrual pain	59

Microorganisms	66
Microwave	15
Moisturizing action	61,62
Molecular size	33
MRSA	52,57
Muscle and joint pain	22,23,34,37,43,46,65
Myrrh	16,22,31,54,55,58-59,73,74,76,78,93
Neurotransmitter	47
Nigella	68
Nootkatone	2,16
Nosocomial infection	55,112,118
Odors	8,25,26,27,58,88,90
Olfactory system	26
Olive oil	9,11,36,78,82
Orange	11,22,23,28,51,54
Oregano (origanum)	3,22,35,45,54,57
Organic plants	4,5,10,62
Organic chemistry	2
Pain	21,26,43-48,59
Pathogens	24,33,51,52,66,105-111,114,119
Peppermint oil	23,40
Perfume	1,4,9,16,22,25,26,34,49,54,58,59,85-91,93
Pesticide	4,5,10
Phytochemicals	68
Phytomedicine	19,52,57
Phytotherapy	53
Pomade	12
Pores	33,37
Probiotics	24,51,105,108,114
Purity	2,9,10,16,27,29,35,56,66,81,83,85,87,105
QOL	26,57
Respiratory problems	19,21,22,27,34,110
Rose oil	*See Attar of Roses*
Rosemary	22,30,35,39,40,54
Sage	21,22,30,35,39,52,54

NOTES